MW01490321

Chapter Titles

Dedication

I dedicate this book to my wonderful sister, Debbie, who always inspires me, teaches me, encourages me, and loves me unconditionally.

I also dedicate this book to all of the nurses and healthcare personnel who have given their heart and soul in caring for humanity.

My Journey

This is the day. This is the moment in time when I start writing a book written by ME.

Writing a book about the funny aspects of my long nursing career has been percolating in my mind for many years. In fact, I even have a file in my office entitled **The Lighter Side.** The file contains historical info, anecdotes, jokes, and stories from my career that I have jotted down for close to 40 years. You see, for the length of my career, when something funny or outrageous happened, I would state aloud, "Well that event made my book."

I have kept that file close to me, in a locked cabinet, like a time capsule, stored away, knowing that someday I would open up that file and look at it in anticipation. I would take my time and read each page carefully. I would savor its contents. I was certain that it would evoke tears: tears of laughter, of sadness, of memories. It was time. It was time to open up that file.

I had a plan: I would write a book. The book would be heartfelt, funny, silly, and lighthearted. Stories would pour out of my soul. I would interject my own feelings, opinions, and views on issues within the healthcare realm. I would be free to say exactly what I wanted to say because, after all, it would be MY book.

And so, the time is now. I have so many ideas whirling around in my brain. I can't wait to see the stories in print. I am excited to get started.

And so, I offer up this book to the world, especially to every last one of us who passionately worked or still works in the greatest, most essential profession of earth: **NURSING.**

And so, LET'S GOOOO!

Disclaimer

Helloooo to my readers. Welcome to my book, the book that I wrote, filled with my experiences. It is my story. They are my tales to tell. They are my thoughts. This book is filled with my crazy sense of humor. It is my reality.

All names have been changed. Had to. No exact locations that I have worked at will be stated, for fear of someone sending me a nasty note or spitting on me.

You may think that a particular situation mentioned is one that you were part of. That is because life repeats itself and crazy situations happen over and over again. Or maybe you were part of it. Don't worry. I won't single you out. At least I won't say your real name out loud.

I may seem disgruntled or frustrated at times in these writings. That is because those of us who are passionate about the medical profession are disturbed by what is going on inside of healthcare, right now. I have watched it slowly go downhill, and that saddens me tremendously.

While I compose this book, I do NOT intend to offend anyone or any group, even though I probably do. I will be laughing with you and not at you. At least that is what I am claiming.

This book is simply loaded with my funny, odd, and unique experiences that are retold as close to reality as possible. The quotes are exactly as I remember them. Keep in mind that I am in my 60's. Thank God that I had foresight and wrote down most of the incidents shortly after they happened.

So, may I invite you to sit back, get a cup of coffee, tea, beer, wine, pineapple juice, or whatever you like and are allowed to drink, and enjoy reading this book as much as I did writing it.

Here Goes

If you get offended easily, please DO NOT read this book because it will upset you. If you despise Ricky Gervais's sense of humor, this book ain't for you. If Chris Rock or the ol' Don Rickles make your blood boil, please return this book, and definitely don't read it or share it with people like YOU.

If you are looking for factual and researched medical information, you are about to read the wrong prose. Everything written in this book reflects only my discoveries and experiences in a comical format. They are my thoughts and summations. Need facts? May I suggest that you don't watch the news, but rather go to the library. Look for medical facts there. Medical websites also hold healthcare facts, but you have to search for them. However:

If silliness, sarcasm, and socially-unacceptable humor are what you seek, well then read on. If you are a nurse, a medical professional, or someone who simply enjoys healthcare stories, you've hit the jackpot. If you want to laugh until you cry, smile with understanding, and commiserate with a crusty old nurse, then this is the book for you. If you find healthcare very confusing, then you may find my answers to why in this book. Also, if you find aspects of medicine that make you shake your head, well than, buy this book and buy one for all of your family members and friends. It will bring light to the craziness.

If you have ever worked in the hospital healthcare industry, may I dare say, YOU WILL LOVE THIS BOOK. I not only wrote it for me but also for you, too. After all, we have put up with soooo much shit, figuratively and literally speaking. Our only coping mechanism for survival in medicine has been laughter. We are able to experience the most horrific situations, and then by some tweaked, weird-ass means, we have been able to find humor in that situation. In short, it is either laugh or curl up into a ball and cry for days.

Every healthcare professional can agree that no one can possibly understand what goes on in our world. You have to live it, breath it, and sit in it to "get it."

And so, I formally invite you to read and enjoy Laughter and Lessons: Healthcare Stories from a Nurse, by ME.

My Story

At age 17, I graduated from high school and took a year-long dental assisting certification class. Out of that program, I immediately got a job with the best dentist on this planet. He had just graduated from Northwestern University with his dental degree, so we puppies working together were a perfect match. By the way, he was also the best boss that I've ever had. We still keep in touch.

After working as a dental assistant for a year, I was hungry for more education. I was struggling with my decision on what career path to follow: dental hygiene or nursing. Fortunately, I was blessed to find out that both programs had the same prerequisites.

And so, I enrolled at a local junior college and began whittling away at the requirements, by taking two, three credit classes a semester while still working at the dental office in order to afford life.

After my prerequisites were completed, I applied to dental hygiene and nursing programs. As luck and hard work would have it, I was accepted into both. I decided to attempt the nursing program first and if I didn't like it, I would still be able to apply to the dental hygiene program the following semester.

I began the BSN program at a wonderful university and never looked back. I had a fantastic education that took me 10 years to pay back, but it was worth every cent.

I would be remiss if I didn't discuss "the wind beneath my wings" during nursing school and for years following my graduation (and honestly, even now): my sister, Debbie. One paragraph is definitely not enough to show my gratitude. She not only encouraged me emotionally and psychologically, but she supported me financially as well. My sister let me stay with her for pennies, and I mean cents. I would have never been able to afford life, let alone pay for an expensive private university education without her support in every way. I am forever indebted to her. (BTW: This wonderful sister of mine is not only a retired teacher, after dealing with teenagers for around 41 years, OMG, but she also writes children's books. Check it out at Debonair Books).

My nursing career started in Florida in early 1982.

In 1982, during my last year of nursing school, we were able to test for our LPN, or licensed practical nurse (LVN on the West Coast). I passed the test and immediately started working on a trauma/pre-post op, 57-bed unit in a hospital in South Florida. I was also still working at the dental office and taking a full load of nursing classes. NO SLEEP FOR ME.

After receiving my Bachelor of Science in Nursing and passing the boards-from-hell, I did a stint at another community hospital for one year. I worked on a med-surg unit that cared for criminally insane humans. (I speak of this in a later chapter.)

After a year of trial by fire, I transferred back to the hospital where I had worked as an LPN. I had only worked on the same trauma/surgery unit for nine months when I was asked to take the charge nurse position on the 3:00-11:00 P. M. shift. "Sure, I said. Sounds fun."

When you are in your 20s, you don't know what you don't know, but you think you know. Make sense?

Let's just call the first three years after nursing school the fastest learning period of my career.

I worked with fantastic nurses, both LPNs and RNs. We labored hard and played hard after work on Miami Beach. "Weeee!"

The 1980s for me, hold great memories and fantastic experiences. I treasure those times.

I stayed at that hospital until the end of 1989, when I became a traveling nurse for the next two and a half years. My travels took me to hospitals in the Western United States. I worked on various units for three to six months, including pre-post-op, orthopedic trauma, ENT/plastic surgery, med-surg, step-down units, etc. I floated in many hospitals to oncology units, pediatrics, post-partum units, heart transplant units, etc.

I ended up taking a permanent job as a charge nurse on a step-down unit, in a wonderful hospital in San Jose, California. I had completed a six-month travel assignment there.

That conversation went something like this:

The Unit Manager: "You are about to leave us for your next travel assignment, right?"

Me: "Yes. I am probably heading to Boston."

Manager: "I would like to offer you a permanent charge nurse position on the day shift. Are you willing to stop traveling?"

Me: "I love travel nursing. I have been able to meet wonderful nurses, see the West, and have fun."

Manager: "But we can offer you full medical coverage, dental coverage, a pension, and $6373.82 per hour. At least it sounded like that to me.

(The East Coast and the West Coast were paid very differently in the '80s and '90s. Unfortunately, I hear that the low pay for nurses still exists in many areas of this country.)

Me: "What? How long do I have to commit to?"

Manager: "One year."

Me: "Let me think about it." Five seconds later: "Ok. I've thought about it. YES. YES. I will do it. I will take the job."

I worked at three different facilities within that HMO hospital system.

In the mid-'90s, I transferred to ER where I stayed until retirement on October 1, 2021.

I am proud to tell you that I worked for the very best HMO in this country, for the final 30 years of my career. This hospital system secured a wonderful pension for me, encouraged growth through a nursing clinical ladder, and offered lateral movement to other units. I am reaping the benefits of devotion and a solid nursing career, now, in retirement.

It took only a few years of nursing to understand why my parents did NOT want me to be a nurse. They were teachers and wanted me to follow that path. They simply wanted to shelter me from the sadness, tragedies, and horrors that I would experience in the nursing profession. I understand.

Yep. I did experience all of those things. But the majority of the time, I helped human beings get better and thrive. There is no better feeling than helping to save a life. I picked the perfect career for me. I love my sisters and brothers who worked alongside me, from doctors and nurses, to x-ray techs, phlebotomists, ER techs, housekeepers, etc. I was very blessed to work with amazing healthcare professionals who also advocated for the wellness of patients.

Tears! I absolutely loved my nursing career, for 1000 reasons. It defined exactly who I was and who I will always be. I am certain that I have fulfilled my destiny. Nursing will forever be one of my greatest passions.

My Mantras and My Words

There are words and phrases that I have used over and over throughout my 40-year nursing career. I still use them in retirement.

I used this verbiage so often at my job, that other staff members referred to them as "Robinisms." They caught on. I even heard other nurses using my little ditties. They seem to be relevant in healthcare.

They are my personal mantras. They are my words that I made up, created new definitions to, or just borrowed to use prn (as needed). Get to know them as I use them throughout this book.

My Mantras:

There is always ONE. …or should I say, at least ONE. They exist in every family, job, neighborhood, class, and society. They are dropped by aliens to simply ruin your day and your life. They cause havoc. They cause discord. They irritate the heck out of everyone.

Don't wish them gone, for when they leave, a new one always appears. You will have to begin all over again, learning how to avoid, ignore, and deal with these fleas.

I'm on the wrong planet. This planet keeps getting weirder and weirder. I beg for the spaceship to land and take me home. I declared this daily in the hospital, and I still do, now, in society in general.

My theory: Do you wonder why, "I Mated with an Alien from Another Planet," is no longer on the cover of tabloids? It's because aliens know that this planet's inhabitants are nuts. They probably refuse to return, let alone have sex with us.

George Bernard Shaw said, "The longer I live, the more convinced I am that this planet is used by other planets as a lunatic asylum."

Exactly!

Send the mail to the right address. Nurses, although angels, are not responsible for EVERYTHING, once you enter into a medical facility. Each employee in a hospital has responsibilities dictated by a job description.

Yet, I have been yelled at for the awful hospital food; how long it takes to obtain lab results; why a doctor has not shown up in the room yet; for the bleach-smelling sheets; for the weather; for the temperature in the hospital, etc.

There is an appropriate address for each of the above complaints and ALL COMPLAINTS, in general. For example:

Food? Talk to the dietitian or cafeteria. I have absolutely no responsibility for the food in this hospital or any other hospital for that matter. Trust me. If I were in charge of food, Gordon Ramsey would be the caterer.

Lab times? I have devoted a whole section of this book to the lab. Write a complaint letter or call them directly. I have done so on many, many occasions.

Where is the doctor? Let me break it to you: They are ridiculously busy and you are not the only one here. I promise you that they are NOT lost or sitting around reading the newspaper. There is a method to their madness. They head to the really critical patients first. Sorry. This is not like your doctor's office where you have an appointment time.

The Temperature in the Hospital? Give it up. I have been fighting that fight for years. I would wear three layers of clothes IN THE SUMMER while working in the hospital. And no, the 58-degree temperature does NOT kill germs.

It just makes us nurses keep going back and forth to the blanket warmer to obtain warm blankets for our freezing patients and for ourselves.

To summarize: Nurses have no control over anything but nursing, and even that applies only some of the time. We are often stuck in the middle and being pulled in 10 directions. We seem to be EVERYBODY'S address. Needless to say, if you have a gripe, then we can direct you to the correct one, and we will.

We are all in this war together! …and it sure is a war. We are fighting a battle in healthcare every single day, against germs, evil, misinformation, tragedy and despair. The thing is, we all need to work together to win that war. We need to be on the same team. None of us stand alone. So just remember: We are all fighting the SAME WAR.

Weeeeeeeeee! My favorite mantra. I use it all the time to express glee and excitement. You wouldn't think that "weeee" would have its place inside a hospital or ER, but it does.

i.e. You finally get test results back after waiting for, what seemed to be, days. =Weeeee!

The 25-year-old patient's cancer screening recheck has come back negative=Weeeee! And hallelujah as well.

Someone ordered lunch for the entire staff, and you actually have time to eat it=Weeeee!

It is 3:15 P.M. and it's time to go home from a long, busy day, working in the ER=Weeeee!

You don't know what you don't know, but you think you know, which makes you dangerous.

During my career as a nurse, I precepted/trained nurses, EMT's, paramedics, and high school students deciding if nursing was a good fit for them.

I would tell my students, "You don't know what you don't know. You become dangerous if you think you know and act on it. Guessing can hurt someone. Please say, "I don't know," if you don't know. I will show you."

That kept everyone safe.

…and last, but not least by far:

Treat all patients like they are your mother, providing you love your mother!

I will try to type here without getting emotional and dropping tears on my computer:

I had the greatest mother who ever existed in this universe. She was beautiful, inside and out, and she was loving, kind, selfless, considerate, affectionate, smart, giving, etc. etc. etc.

I remember when she had absolutely NO $. I was in my senior year of high school. My parents were divorced. I was living with her. We were watching TV when one of those ads came on for the Red Cross or one of those organizations.

The TV screen was filled with malnourished, bony, kids. My mother opened her dresser drawer, pulled out two one-dollar bills, and mailed that money away to that organization.

That event, and so many more things that I witnessed my mother do, taught me how to treat humanity. "Treat others the way you want to be treated." My mother preached it, taught it, said it, and lived by it every day.

This mantra was injected into me by my mother.

My Words:

Why should Daniel Webster have the market on words? Anyone should be able to come up with their own words and/or definitions. I stand for freedom of expression, which includes the birth of words and their meanings. I am certain that you have a few made up words of your own.

Here are some of mine:

Cheecha: Pronounced Chee + cha (like the cha in chacha)

All of my "cheechas" are smiling right now, as they read this. I still use this word quite frequently.

The word was born in the year 2000, when I adopted a beautiful red Doberman puppy, named Athena. She was the sweetest pup ever. I called her my little chee chee initially, which ultimately turned into Cheecha. I rarely called her Athena after that word was created.

It is a term of endearment. It has come to mean cute things, sweet kids and pets, and lovely friends and coworkers. It also became my name as used by a few nurses who I worked with.

I added a few spinoffs of Cheecha:

Cheezit: A cheezit is a cute, young animal or child.

Chee Chee: A small thing, or in plural form, means breasts.

There is an actual word in the dictionary, Chicha, which means a fermented beverage.

Nee nee: Pronounced knee knee.

I think that a boyfriend of mine threw this word out into the air when I was in my 20s, and I caught it. I don't remember exactly what his definition was, but I believe it was close to this.

My definition of a nee nee is some kind of growth on your body. It could be, for example, a skin tag, a mole, a wart or a freckle. It is a nicer and cuter way to describe a foreign body living on your skin, I think.

Incidentally, a nene is actually an endangered goose. (I changed the spelling as well).

Hoo ha: Pronounced as written.

Funny enough, I thought that I made this definition up, but apparently, I didn't. Listed in the Urban Dictionary, hoo ha is a non-offensive term for a woman's vagina.

Hoo-ha actually means to exclaim in surprise or a condition of excitement according to Mr. Webster.

I'm certain that you could come up with a funny correlation between Webster's definition and the urban one.

Choo Chee: Also pronounced as written.

My definition is any male or female private part, below the waist.

Interestingly enough, I have used hoo ha and choo chee in explaining a patient's problem to another healthcare professional. In context, people seem to understand my meaning without question.

In reality, choo chee is a curry dish. It is a thick, red, Thai curry made with seafood. Another spelling, chu chi, is "to feel jealous" in Chinese.

These mantras and words were used by me daily, in my medical career, at home, and everywhere I went, for that matter. They helped me survive and thrive. I still use all of them, as you will note while reading this book.

And so, the moral of this chapter is, go on and make up your own verbiage, or use mine. What's the worst that could happen?

A+B=C

I usually look at life as a glass of juice that is mostly full. Because of this quality of mine, I have tried to make sense of all the college courses that I was required to take to achieve a Bachelor of Science in Nursing. On my educational journey, I often asked myself, "What was the point in learning stuff that I would never use in my career or anywhere else for that matter?" All classes HAD to have a purpose. Turns out they did, just not for the obvious ones.

For example, microbiology.

One would think that this class for a person entering the medical profession was one of the most important classes to take. After all, bugs and medicine go hand in hand. Right?

I know now that most of that micro class has little to do with what I do as a bedside nurse. Microbes are for the lab, doctors, and the housekeepers to deal with, not this ED nurse.

Healthcare professionals are taught to wash their hands or use hand sanitizer until their skin flakes off. We do, and it does.

Today, good hand washing seems to be the answer to destroying bugs. I didn't need a semester class to know that fact.

OK. Nurses do need to know about just a few bugs: the ones that cause our patients to get very sick, for example, and especially the ones that cause nurses to sneeze repeatedly and miss work and feel bad. The rest of the bugs are dealt with by other hospital workers, specifically the doctors.

I have, however, found a huge use for that micro class:

I thought my teacher for microbiology was the worst teacher ever. I now appreciate her.

My microbiology instructor would start the class by taking roll. She would yell out what pages to read, and leave the room for the remainder of class time. This went on for the entire three-credit college course, including the final exam.

Due to my eagerness to learn, and the fact that my parents were teachers, accompanied by my unrealistic belief, at age 24, that all things in college classes were important, I did read all the material. Fortunately, I learned not only about the bugs/germs that cause us to cough and sneeze, but also about the ingredients and recipes for making beer and wine. "Weeeee!"

Today, viruses and bacteria are much, much less important to my life than beer and wine-tasting weekends in Amador County, California. And so yes, I DID need microbiology. Who knew?

Next case in point: algebra? What the….

Who really cares about A or B or even C for that matter? Would an algebra equation ever determine if my patient should go on life-support or not?

What I am trying to say is that for many years, I had absolutely no recognizable use for Algebra 1, Algebra 2 or Algebra 10 for that matter. I had no use for that info while I was taking the class and no use until…

Drum roll please.

May 15, 2015. As I was in the midst of caring for a 380 lb., 50-year-old female patient, it came to me. I gasped. Algebra actually made sense to me. Like a bolt of lightning, A+B=C! Why yes, it does.

Examples:

#1 A 5 foot, 2-inch-tall, 50-year-old female, that weighs 380 pounds + two knees that have been holding her up for the past 50 years = sore knees and "I can't walk."

Eureka! A+B=C

#2 A 2+ pack-a-day male smoker for 50 years + "I can't breathe" =COPD (Chronic Obstructive Pulmonary Disease)

This is a wonderful discovery.

#3 A 55-year-old male who confesses to drinking beer since the age of 15 + tells me that his wife left him and she won't let him see his children = depression and suicidal ideations.

Algebra has become meaningful.

#4 A 35-year-old male who doesn't work and has a body covered in tattoos and piercings + he admits to smoking meth every day, thanks to his $ from disability + he states that he is having chest pain = rapid heart rate, at the very least.

Don't get me started or you will learn my political affiliation.

See how easy it is to understand medicine simply by applying ALGEBRA. Who knew?

And last, but certainly not least, let's discuss my one-credit class on Florence Nightingale. Here I was, working two jobs to afford college and taking a full load of classes. That one-credit class was mandatory. It was only offered at 3:00 P.M. Are you kidding me? I had to leave work early once a week to hear about "The Lady with the Lamp?" or my version: "The Lady and the Tramps."

Couldn't we have summed up Flo's life in 10 minutes during the med-surg class?

Surprise. This class provided some of the most meaningful content of my education.

It took me 30 years to appreciate Florence.

Here is what I remember and now appreciate about this amazing advocate of our profession:

-She was born in the first part of the 1800s to a wealthy/privileged English family, but she chose to care for the sick and injured. (Say what? She definitely had a calling.)

-Several men courted her and asked for her hand in marriage, but she never wanted to get married, and so she didn't. (You go on with your bad self, sister.)

-Nursing was for those of "ill-repute" in those days. That didn't bother old Flo. (Equal opportunity employer).

-Nursing was self-taught for Florence. She also used a ton of common sense in her approach to patient care and healthcare reforms. (A lost approach nowadays).

-In 1854 or so, the Crimean War started with Britain/France vs. the Russians. An army hospital was set up in Scutari, India.

-Hospitals were ill-equipped and poorly staffed at that time.

Patients were lined up in the hallways, and every bed was taken. (Boy, things have changed. Not!)

-Florence organized a pool of 40 "ladies" to care for about 18,000 injured soldiers. (Glad the patient-nurse ratio has changed slightly.)

-Florence began implementing proper hygiene and sanitation when she saw that dirty rags were used as dressings for wounds, there was a cholera outbreak in the hospital, and rats were everywhere. (Took a nurse to notice?) And of course, after a nurse took over, the mortality rate went down.

-She financed a lot of changes with her own $. (Impressive).

-One of my favorite things that I learned about Florence Nightingale was that she worked side-by-side with the other nurses. Every night, she would check in on patients, for morale reasons, while holding a lamp to light the way.
A London newspaper article dubbed her "The Lady with the Lamp." (Did she ever sleep? Sounds about right for nurses even today).

In short, Flo pioneered nursing and hospital reforms, campaigned for sanitation and cleanliness, founded the first nursing school, promoted the well-being of soldiers, and performed a ton more incredible acts.

Florence Nightingale lived an amazing life and died at age 90 of heart failure. (I just looked that up).

Wow. Why was that class only one credit? Why was Algebra three credits? It shall remain a mystery.

And so, in conclusion, regarding the multitude of classes I was required to take, they all had a purpose, apparently.

It just took time and effort for me to figure this out.

To make nurses who graduated with a BSN feel like they'd climbed Mt. Everest (which is probably easier than nursing school as the climb takes less time, less money, and less oxygen), **The Guinness Book of World Records** posted the following on May 18, 2011:

The Bachelor of Science in Nursing (BSN) degree has been chosen as the toughest degree among all the undergraduate college degrees.

It has 64 university exams, 130 series exams and 174 assignments within 4 years.

Definitely felt like more.

Triage

Triage: A preliminary assessment of patients in order to decide the urgency of the situation. That is it, in a nutshell.

In the ER, a crucial decision is made the second a patient walks in. "How serious is this complaint? Do I have time to "fiddle around" or does this person need immediate attention? What does this person actually need? How soon do they need it?"

It is as simple as that.

There are protocols that determine the level of urgency. They go something like this:

Level 1: CPR in progress: Holy Crap! Nurses' and doctors' adrenalin is flowing like water out of the Sierra Nevada Mountain Range in April. (i.e., cardiopulmonary arrest)

Level 2: Better hurry up and do something or CPR will be needed. (i.e., respiratory distress)

Level 3: No life-threatening disabilities as of yet. More to come. The patient has a bit of time, hopefully. (i.e., abdominal pain, headache)

Level 4: Ok. Take a seat. We will be with you in a bit. (i.e., sore throat for the past 20 minutes)

Level 5: WTF? This couldn't wait until you see or talk to your primary doctor? You came to our seriously-overcrowded ER with an average of a four to six-hour wait today for this? (i.e., "I need a letter for my companion cat so that I don't get evicted.")

The following tales are just a few of my experiences as a triage nurse. Other triage stories are scattered throughout this book. They are real stories, people. I hope they make you laugh.

Here is a funny triage story. It's cute, but my family and friends think there is no better tale. They think it is the best story ever. I have told approximately 56,982 work stories: happy ones, funny ones, a few sad ones, etc.

But for some reason, this is the only one that family and friends ever reference. In actuality, I am pretty sure that they don't even remember any other ones.

And so, to make all of my non-medical friends and family happy, here is their favorite triage story, EVERRRRRR!

It was 8:00 A.M. I was in triage with one other nurse. In walks a young couple in their early 30s with their five-year-old boy. On the triage paperwork, yes, it was before computers, under the reason for the visit, it said, "five-year-old with penis injury."

The mother sat down in a chair next to me with Noah on her lap. Noah looked like any happy five-year-old boy holding a toy army man. The father stood next to the mother and son.

I started the conversation with, "Hello. My name is Robin. So, what happened to Noah?"

Noah's mother immediately spoke up and said, "Noah was playing with little, green, plastic army men while he was trying to pee. The lid was up on the toilet. One of the army men fell into the toilet. Noah grabbed the lid to steady himself so that he could reach into the toilet for the army man. The lid fell onto his penis. I think I saw a little blood on the end of it. I just want to make sure that he is ok."

Ok. Easy enough, right?

I said to Noah, "Hi Noah. I am Robin the nurse. Can you please stand up and slip your pants down so that I can check your penis?" Noah jumped up, facing me, and pulled his pants down. I then said, "Noah, I am going to touch your penis and look at it for a few seconds to make sure it is not injured or hurt."

Noah's reply:

"Sure, go ahead. And it feels really good if you pull on it, too!"

Dad immediately yelled, "That's my boy."

Mom simultaneously stated, "Noah, don't say that."

I exited stage left, holding back my hysterical laughter until I was located far away from any humans.

I did return after a minute, composed I may add.

Noah's penis was unscathed.

This initial complaint could have been a triage level 2, but it wasn't. Noah was seen in the triage area by our ED doctor who said, "You're fine Noah. Go home and play with your army men. And Dad, you better give the sex talk now."

Some more triage stories:

A young lady arrived in triage. Her complaint was slight vaginal pain from "accidentally sitting on a big decorative light bulb." Ouch. I opted to not ask her for the real story. I also opted to let the doctor explain why a large light bulb would need to have an outboard motor attached to it, in order to make its way up the vagina.

FYI, she was a level 3. She had a small vaginal laceration.

Please people, get a hobby!

Next:

A middle-aged male arrived, rather stumbled, into the triage chair. He reeked of alcohol. My bias, or rather experience, said that he was definitely intoxicated.

I knew that part of his diagnosis would be alcohol abuse. Concerns floated around in my head: Did he drive here? Hopefully not. He would obviously need the social worker or discharge planner to help him secure treatment for alcoholism or, at the very least, he'd need a ride home, at some point.

I began the questioning:

Me: "Hello sir. How can I help you."

Mr. Pickled: "I need to let you know that I am planning on setting the world on fire. This world is a mess. The world has gone crazy. We need to start from scratch. I am annoyed at what is happening in it right now."

Me: Thinking to myself: "Well, he is one of the sanest human beings that I have had contact with all day." (Kidding. There were others.) I immediately found him a room in our psych area and gave the nurse and doctor a "heads up."

Onward:

This is what healthcare professionals have to deal with:

A 40ish year-old man was pacing in the waiting room. It was his turn. I called him into my triage area. This is close to how it went:

Me: Hello. "My name is Robin. You are welcome to take a seat. What can I do for you on this lovely day?"

Mr. Meth Head: (Pacing in the triage area looking frantic) "Quick. I need an enema to remove the meth that I shoved up my ass."

Me: Ugh....

I don't remember what happened after that.

Our mind is a wonderful thing. Sometimes, it blocks fine details to an event, that it doesn't want us to remember. Sometimes it shuts out the entire thing. It protects our souls.

Other times, for me, crappy things come flooding back into my brain at 3:00 A.M., which is my personal bewitching hour.

Next:

I had just finished triaging a 30-something-year-old male.

Me: "Ok sir. You can have a seat in the waiting room. Your name will be called when a bed is available."

Let's call this gent Fabio.

Fabio: "Um. How long is this going to take?"

Me: "Not sure. It depends on what comes in the back door." (Ambulance traffic).

Fabio: "Do you have any girlie magazines? If I have to wait, can you get me some girlie magazines?"

Me: Orangutan stare. Pausing. Giving him a chance to retract his request. "What?"

Fabio: Obviously slightly irritated. "Do you have any "Playboy" or "Penthouse" magazines that I can look at while I am waiting? I need something to do."

I handed him a "Good Housekeeping" and a "Sports Illustrated", outdated issues. Sorry. All that we had.

… last triage story, in this chapter.

It was early in the morning.

An elderly woman in her 80s, using a cane, arrived in my triage area. She had a slight limp. I invited her to sit down in the chair next to the desk. Her daughter was with her.

Here is pretty much what happened:

Me: "Hello, my sweet. My name is Robin. What brings you to the ER?"

Lovely woman. We shall call her Mildred. She looked like a Mildred.

Mildred: "I was wearing the wrong shoes. I slipped and fell and now my right hip hurts. I can still walk, but it's sore. There is no mark or anything."

Me: "Did you land on the rug, tile, or the ground?"

Mildred: "No. I slipped and my hip hit hard against the organ in our living room. Then I sat down on the floor. My husband helped me up."

I completed a quick assessment.

Me: "Ok, Mildred. I am going to get the doctor. He will examine you and then will determine what x-rays we need to do."

Mildred: "Thank you so very much. I didn't want to come here but my daughter made me."

Me: "Of course, she did. She wants the best for you, Mildred. She wants to make sure that you don't have any major injuries."

An aside: I love the elderly. They are my favorite age group. The other nurses who I worked with, knew this about me. They would occasionally state, "I have your patient, Robin, in room 10. He is the cutest little old man."

I even told my charge nurse "I am confining my practice to those people who are elderly war veterans." After all, they only show up in the ER with actual emergencies. They are kind and appreciative as well. My request was denied.

The older population usually has to be dragged into the hospital or a relative would have had to call 911, appropriately.

Onward:

I went to the doctor's office and reviewed the case with a doctor. He came out to the triage area, introduced himself and examined Mildred. As he was walking away, he stated, "I will put the order in for the X-ray."

I obtained a wheelchair and brought Mildred over to the X-ray department. I left her in line and went to tell the X-ray techs that "Mildred" was waiting for her X-ray:

Me: "Hi, gang. I have Mildred here from triage, right outside this door. She is in her 80s with a right hip injury. Her daughter is with her."

X-ray Techs: Five or so, of them. Hysterically laughing.

Me: "What's up? Do I have something on my face?"

X-ray Tech: One of the techs finally stopped laughing long enough and pointed to the order, which read:

Patient Fell onto Husband's Organ

"9-1-1.

What Is Your Emergency?"

I have so many things to say on this subject. I really don't know where to begin. I am sure that you can imagine, though. After all, 40 years in healthcare lends itself to lots and lots of wild and crazy stories and fodder for my book, especially when 3/4 of my nursing career was spent working in emergency services.

Let's start from the very beginning: Why call 9-1-1?

9-1-1 was designated to be used for EMERGENCIES ONLY, in the U.S.A. It was designed as a way for the public to gain fast and easy access to care in an emergent situation. Let me repeat that: EMERGENT SITUATION.

I contend that I am on the wrong planet. And so, on the planet that I hope to be heading to soon, when you call 9-1-1, you must first define the word "EMERGENCY", and then let the operator know how your situation fits into that word. If they find it in their protocol, you get to ride free.

Don't you worry. There are a million protocols everywhere these days. If your complaint does not fall into any of their protocols, ding ding, then it is NOT an emergency, and you can go on with your day and so can the rest of us. You are welcome to find another avenue to solve your issue.

For the sake of 9-1-1 and EVERYONE, an emergency is defined as:

-Any type of fire, in a building or car for example.

-Any serious medical problem like a seizure, chest pain, or hemorrhage.

-Any life-threatening situation like a fight with a person with a weapon (happening wayyyy too often these days).

-A way to report a crime in progress.

And:

-If you have a rattlesnake in your wood pile. What the heck? Do they have a protocol for removing snakes at the 9-1-1 office? Shocking.

Side note:

Trust me. I did not initially believe this myself. Go ahead and feel free to laugh on my account, as I ramble on about my use of 9-1-1 "appropriately." Who knew?

I was ignorant and did not know that my city's fire department handles snakes as well as life-threatening emergencies. You heard me right. 9-1-1 takes care of vermin in my town.

I found a large, alive, and hissing, rattlesnake in my wood pile. Truth be told, my female Doberman, Xenia, found it. I heard her barking and barking and barking. (FYI: Dobermans don't bark unless there is actually an issue.) I was forced to check out the reason for the barking. Yep, she had a darn good reason for alerting me.

I called Animal Control and the conversation went something like this:

Me: "What? You want me to call 9-1-1 for a snake? Don't those kind souls have more important things to do?"

Lady at animal control: "Ma'am. That is what they do in our county."

Me: "Okie Dokie. Seems like a waste of valuable resources."

Lady at animal control: "Ma'am, rattlesnakes are poisonous."

Me: "I got it."

The next phone call occurred like this:

9-1-1 lady: "9-1-1. What is your emergency?"

Me: "Rattlesnake in my woodpile." I'm not sure why, but I was laughing uncontrollably. Still seems like the wrong address for a snake issue.

…and so…

The fire department guys showed up quickly and they were very willing to send their rookie over to the wood pile to dismantle it, find the snake, and kill the rattler as the rest of them stared and chatted with me, while I stood there in my way-too-short, shorts. It was summer. I was single and alone. This was an unexpected event. My focus at the time of the phone call was on the snake, and not on what I was wearing. I swear. Lesson learned.

I am proud that I did not insist that they transport me to the emergency room, but I still felt guilty for utilizing 9-1-1 for a critter removal or rather kill.

In reality, however, people call 9-1-1 for a plethora of reasons, many of which include issues other than emergent care.

According to me, the population in the United States thinks that there are 63,672 reasons to call 911. This is just my estimate. (FYI, most of those complaints do NOT fall under the category of emergent.)

Here are some of my favorites, rather ridiculous, in my opinion, 9-1-1 calls from patients that were delivered to me in the ER:

1. Her husband was using the car and she needed transport to the ER to check out her very, very minor problem. (I don't remember the problem because it was very minor.) Oh yeah…and a taxi or Uber costs $$, but the ambulance is free under their insurance.

My thoughts: She arrived at the ER talking on the phone and was irritated that I, too, needed to speak with her now. And that is why insurance costs are out of control.

2. It was 5:00 P.M. Traffic "was terrible at that hour." Why not call 9-1-1 and have them put their sirens on so that she could jet to the hospital for her sore throat that started 30 minutes prior to her emergent call to 9-1-1?

My thoughts: I swear this happened. No other complaints were offered. She lived to be "entitled" for another day.

3. "I can't walk. I think that I hurt my leg."

My thoughts: Per medics, the patient was walking all over her home, frantically trying to find her purse, without any notable issue, and talking on the phone and telling her friend how she couldn't walk.

My thoughts: Sigh…

4. "A stomach ache just started today after eating" (enough spicy Mexican food for 100 people). "It hurts too much to drive."

My thoughts: Arrives to the ER on the gurney, texting and smiling. He hops off the gurney and climbs onto the hallway bed without missing a beat in no apparent distress whatsoever.

Yes, hallway bed. Nope, he didn't even try an antacid at his house. Yes, we cured him with an antacid; an **emergent** antacid; no different than your home antacid.

5. "I think I have a cold or the flu." Symptoms (stuffy nose, sore throat) started 20 minutes prior to calling 9-1-1.

My thoughts: She lived.

6. "I was short of breath for a few seconds, yesterday. Not today. I feel fine now, but I just want to get checked out."

My thoughts: What does she want us to do? She has no symptoms.

Yes, she was diagnosed as "just fine" and sent home.

7. "I feel stressed."

My thoughts: So, does the entire population living in the USA. Better build a bigger ER. And certainly, you can't drive if you are stressed because driving is stressful and so driving will just make matters worse.

What the heck has happened to civilization?

8. "I know this is not an emergency, but I called 9-1-1 so that I can be put right into a room and get seen right away by a doctor and I don't have to wait. It is my turn to pick the kids up from school, so I need to be out of here in the next hour."

My thoughts: I cannot repeat to you what the overwhelmed brilliant ER physician said when I reported to him what the patient told me.

9. "I got my period early."

My thoughts: I got nothing.

10. A woman sent her teenager in due to "a difficult temperament."

My thoughts: Is there any teenager with a "less-than-difficult" temperament? If so, they deserve an Academy Award for best performance.

11. "Itchy eyes for six months."

My thoughts: We all have itchy eyes from March thru August, and we still drive. That warrants an ambulance ride when you have been driving for the past 6 months? Good God!

12. 24-year-old with pain in the left ear and "I demand a CT scan to make sure that I don't have an aneurysm. I read on Google that it could be an aneurysm and it could kill me."

My thoughts: I got nothing.

13. "I have been getting hot flashes," says a 55-year-old female.

My thoughts: Boy oh boy! If all females called 9-1-1 for all of their hot flashes, then we would need the population of Asia to begin paramedic training immediately.

14. An adult with "Clear goop in my right eye."

My thoughts: Can you see? Yes? What the heck? You can drive but you didn't feel like driving today? Please, aliens from another planet, come and get me.

I have lost faith in humanity. I was raised in the Kennedy era when we lived by, "Ask not what your country can do for you; ask what you can do for your country." I was taught to do unto others as you would want done to you. I was taught to understand the effects of your actions on your neighbors and the world, for that matter. I lived by the idea that we are all in this war together. I am absolutely proud to have been raised in those hard times.

So much of society has become entitled. It is spreading like a wildfire. It is a pandemic that will ultimately destroy us all.

Let me paint this next picture for you:

15. I was heading to the medication room when I heard a nurse yell, "Help!" A patient had passed out and was not breathing. The entire staff in the area ran into the room, me included. Life-saving measures were initiated.

A doctor asked me for something. Sorry, I don't remember what it was.

I was running out of the room to obtain it when I saw a lady walking quickly towards me, fully dressed. I initially thought she was a visitor.

I stepped aside to avoid the woman coming at me. She grabbed my arm.

This "rotten" lady could see the mayhem that was ensuing in the room next to both of us. She saw me urgently heading "somewhere," but she opted to grab me and stop me in my tracks.

This is what occurred:

Rotten Lady: "How much longer 'till I see a doctor? I have been waiting for over 30 minutes," she said while holding on to my arm for dear life.

Me: "I am sorry, but I can't address your issue right this minute as I am with a critical patient." I wiggled my arm free from her death grip.

Rotten Lady: "What? My needs are not important? I am critical too. 9-1-1 brought me here."

This rotten lady saw the events taking place. Did she care about the woman who the staff was trying to revive? Nope. Too entitled.

Rest assured; I have hundreds of more stories. She and all of the other people who call 9-1-1 for erroneous reasons, make it difficult for medical personnel to provide the care needed to critical patients.

Those "rotten eggs" are a cog in the emergency services wheel. They are a speed bump in the road of the ER. They are an annoying splinter in the palm of your right hand when you are right-handed.

Rotten eggs think only about themselves. They don't care that their behaviors ultimately affect us all.

Emergency service people want to help you, but only if you really need it.

Unfounded emergent complaints take time away from the care of actual emergencies.

I can't stress that enough. I lived it, breathed it, experienced it, and swallowed it for years.

All of the peeps who respond to the 9-1-1 calls are heroes! They head to unknown situations, deal with filthy environments, come in contact with horrible, nasty, rotten humans, and amazingly enough, they don't even quit after years of service.

These heroes have brought me their patients. They still smile. They should really be pissed off at times, especially nowadays, when they wait at the ambulance entrance for hours, as there is nowhere to place their patients: "No room at the inn."

You see, due to the volume of patients utilizing 911 incorrectly + using the ER for all of their medical and dental issues= We have no available beds, or gurneys for that matter, for the humans who REALLY, REALLY need help.

What people don't realize is that someone who is having a massive heart attack at home, has to wait a bit longer for assistance from the 9-1-1 crew, because that lady used the emergency call system to help her to bypass traffic. UGH!

And so, in conclusion:

Emergency medical personnel want to help you, but so do your dentist, dermatologist, medical doctor, GYN, psychiatrist, grocery store clerk, and pharmacist. Please send the mail to the right address. The "right address" is not ALWAYS THE ER.

THE END

Privacy.

Is there such a thing anymore?

When I got out of school, privacy in healthcare did not seem to be an issue. Every patient had their own space inside of a room with a door attached that could and would be closed as needed. Hallways were not used for patient care.

In the 1970s and 1980s the population of this planet was much less. Nurses had room to breathe, work, and function. We lived and worked with "Marcus Welby, MD." If you don't know who that is, watch an episode on YouTube. He was my hero. You will be envious of what my initial work environment looked like.

Due to lots of sex, the population has grown substantially. Too many humans and not enough places to stick them.

I am super happy Elon Musk and Richard Branson are researching other places to rehouse some of you.

Unfortunately, I will be long gone when that happens. I have often begged to be transported to a better planet with saner creatures. It obviously hasn't happened yet. I remain hopeful.

Bottom line: Our planet is getting overcrowded. Humans are multiplying fast. Add to that are our open borders in America. Everyone wants to live in the wonderful US of A.

But healthcare is obviously not able to keep up with the demands of a growing population. Again, we need more "cheechas" in healthcare and more buildings to care for the sick.

We now must utilize any available space to provide patients with healthcare. That means a chair in the waiting room with many other people listening to patients talk to the doctor. That means hallway beds, with nurses and doctors examining the sick and doing things while others watch. The flimsy screens provided are a false bravado.

Speaking for the entire medical population, if I may:

"The lack of privacy is not the fault of healthcare workers. We are doing what we can with the space available."

True dat.

If you have to wait for an actual room in order to be evaluated, in a hospital ER, it will most likely take days instead of hours to be seen and treated.

It's like an overcrowded restaurant, minus the reservation capability. You can wait for a lovely table in the corner or just sit anywhere. The table in the corner will be ready in five hours or you can be seated near the bathroom now.

Humans are not known to enjoy waiting, for anything, let alone for healthcare. And so, patients end up taking what they can get, which amounts, sometimes, to no privacy.

Let's add to the fact that we medical people see naked bodies all day long. I am accustomed to seeing people without their clothes on due to my job. I hate to say this, but nudity doesn't faze me one bit. In fact, a man dressed in a gray suit, turns me on much more than him being naked.

What I mean is that many of us healthcare professionals are unaffected by someone removing their clothes, getting naked, and changing into a hospital gown. We are happy to help them do that without them feeling any shame. We do what we can to make them feel comfortable. We do what we can to protect their privacy.

Even so, we sometimes have to remind ourselves to close the curtain, shut the door, or hold the sheet over the patient because we are actually doing and thinking about approximately 463 tasks at one time (give or take 30). Sorry, but this is true.

Oh, and let me add this to the topic of privacy: A curtain does not hide sounds or smells wafting through and around that curtain. I am truly uncertain about the actual benefits of a hospital green, brown, or 1960s flowered curtain. I suppose that it is capable of hiding some things.

With all of the previous info in mind, here are some of my best privacy or lack thereof stories:

A 40-year-old patient of mine was scheduled to have her gallbladder removed in the morning. Let's just call her Bambi.

I needed to get Bambi ready for an early morning surgery. Pre and post-op teaching were in order. Keep in mind that I was young at the time of this event.

Bambi was in a two-bed room with a curtain serving as a wall between beds.

I had not met this patient yet. I gathered my pamphlets and was heading into the room when I heard loud moaning. I stepped into the room and immediately noted that the elderly lady in bed A, was laughing with the covers pulled up over her head. The curtain only slightly shielded Granny from knowing what was happening on the other side.

I jetted over to bed B, only to find two people naked and having sex. The man was on top of my patient. They immediately stopped the bouncing after they noticed me standing at the end of the bed, in astonishment.

Me: "Hello Bambi. I am Robin your nurse. Is 15 minutes long enough for you to finish your activity? I have some teaching to complete for you."

Husband (I assumed): "Five minutes will work," he said while lying on top of her and twisting his neck to see and address me.

Me: "OK. Sorry for the interruption." Exit stage left.

Speed forward in time. If that scene had happened at the end of my career, I probably would have shouted, "Go on with your bad selves! See you in 20."

Next story:

One of the nicest ER physicians on this planet is the protagonist in this play. We shall name him Dr. Houdini.

This story began all of a sudden. This is how I remember it:

I was working in a 20-bed emergency room when I heard banging on the ambulance bay door. I rushed over, pushed the square, silver button on the wall, and let in a very pregnant woman, sitting in a wheelchair. She was being pushed forward by her scared-looking husband followed by four young children. He had driven his wife and kids to the hospital for obvious reasons.

Background info: Let's call this lady, "The Old Woman in a Shoe." (Mrs. OWIAS, for short.) She was 30ish and this was going to be her fifth child. She was moaning loudly saying, "I have to push! I have to push!"

Most of the ER heard her, and I couldn't be happier about that. Several nurses came running to assist me.

You see, I had very little birthing experience as a nurse, plus I have no children. I definitely wanted four kids, but life didn't work out that way for me. However, several nurses who I worked with, transferred to the ER from the Labor and Delivery unit. And so, whenever a woman came into the ER attempting to spit out a newborn, those angels flew right into the room and took over. They hovered over the patient and cared for her, right out of a scene from heaven. That is how I viewed it anyway.

The angels took over pushing Mrs. OWIAS into a room and undressing her quickly. Several of them were also setting up for the delivery of a "cheezit."

Mrs. OWIAS was my patient. I opted to let "the angels" take over her care, and I got them anything they needed. I had already asked the charge nurse to notify the Labor and Delivery unit of this patient's status. They usually sent several of their nurses over to assist with the birth. Thank GOD.

You see, with the advent of state-of-the-art OB/GYN departments, it is a rare thing to deliver a baby in the ER.

I stood with the husband, just inside the curtain, as the angels positioned the mama in stirrups. Mr. O. was such a gentle soul. Every few minutes, this wonderful man would softly declare, "I love you honey." It was a scene out of a Hallmark movie.

Several other staff members and the patient's four children were mingling around on the other side of the curtain. Of course, they could hear everything going on, and thus looked anxious. Mrs. OWIAS's moans were getting louder, and so I ran to get the doctor. The doctor was talking to another physician and said that he would be "right there in a minute."

I went back to be with the husband. I carefully slipped into the room, avoiding pulling the curtain open at all. Mrs. OWIAS's legs were spread wide open, and the top of an infant's head was in clear view. This baby was attempting to escape from her vagina, at that moment.

All of a sudden, the curtain flew all the way open abruptly, as Dr. Houdini loudly stated to the husband, "Hi. I am Dr. Houdini. Can you see everything ok?"

Seeing the kids looking at their mom's HOO HA in astonishment, and watching everyone else staring into the room, I rushed over and flung the curtain closed while firmly stating, "Dr. Houdini, her husband, the kids, the city, and the entire universe can see everything very clearly now that you opened the privacy curtain!"

Laughter filled the room.

No privacy, at all, in childbirth.

Mrs. OWAIS gave birth immediately after that curtain call, without incident. Baby #5 was 100% perfect, but the other four kids were probably scarred for life.

I will end the privacy chapter with this story. It is definitely one of my favorites. It went something like this:

Three male, ER patients were in a row, lying on their gurneys. Green curtains separated them. The nurses' station was in front of these gentlemen.

A doctor needed to examine patient #3 in that row. Let's call that Dr., Stevie Wonder. You are about to figure out why:

I was sitting at the nurse's station charting, in the days of no computers, minding my own business, when I heard Dr. Wonder say loudly, behind the curtain, "I can't seem to find it."

Patient: "What?" The patient was older than dirt and obviously hard of hearing.

Dr. Wonder: Raising his voice louder: "I can't find it. Do you still have it?"

Patient: "What?"

Dr. Wonder: Screaming now: "I can't locate your penis. Do you still have one?"

Patient: Also yelling: "What? Are you asking me a question?"

Dr. Wonder: Screaming at the top of his lungs: "Do you have a penis? I am having trouble finding it."

Patient: "What?"

I had had enough. All of the patients, visitors, and staff members in our 20-bed ER, were definitely aware that Mr. Older-Than-Dirt had NO VISIBLE PENIS. The two gentlemen in the other beds next door, were chuckling.

I got up from my chair, walked over to the curtain that was supposed to block sound, and said, "Excuse me, Dr. Wonder. I have the ladies from Hooters down the street, on line one. They heard you. They are willing to come over and help you find this man's penis. What should I tell them?"

Needless to say, the laughter was deafening.

Dr. Wonder walked out from behind the curtain with a smile on his face, shaking his head. I stated, "Dr. Wonder, you made my book!"

What is Going on with Healthcare?

Get ready for a rant! This is my most serious and passionate section. I could ramble on and on with most of these issues. You're in luck. I chiseled the subjects way down to just one chapter.

I believe that if you bitch about anything, you should follow it up with a solution or at least a few suggestions for improvement. And so, here goes a ton of bitching with my solutions. Enjoy.

What's happening inside the healthcare system is unacceptable!

My opinion: Healthcare was once a wonderful planet. A human could get excellent medical care in a timely manner. Doctors, nurses, medics, social workers, dietary staff, etc. loved their jobs, and they were treated with utmost respect.

We all focused on our patients 100% of the work day. Healthcare employees were expected to get their patients healthy by using knowledge-based practice. Supplies were abundant. Referrals were easily made to the appropriate specialty.

We all dressed, looked, and acted the part. We had specific roles: Nursing did nursing, respiratory therapy did respiratory, and the lab did lab. Not now.

There was enough room in hospitals and clinics. People did not wait for hours to obtain quality care. Patients stayed in the hospital until they were actually well enough to care for themselves or had help.

Something went awry overnight, or so it seems.

Hospitals have evolved into insane places to visit, check into, or work at. They are extraordinarily busy. I don't mean somewhat busy. I mean there are often more people than that building can fit. ER waiting rooms look like an entrance to a rock concert just before the doors open.

On any given day, many more people need to lie down than there are beds or gurneys, whether it be in the hospital units or the emergency room.

The extraordinarily high patient volume is one of the reasons patients are kicked out of a hospital before they feel that they are ready.

Hospitals are busting at the seams.

Add multiple pandemics to the picture, and you can imagine what healthcare has been like over the last decade.

For starters, the ER was not invented to be a clinic. We definitely want to help you, but we were designed to handle your EMERGENCIES.

Do you have an urgent/emergent concern? We are there for you. Not an emergency? Please consider making an appointment with your doctor or sending your doctor a message filled with your requests. Urgent care clinics have sprouted up all over this country and are available to you as needed. If that doesn't work, "Come on down." ….and wait. We will eventually see you. We have to.

Case in point:

It was a typical Saturday night in the emergency room. The waiting room was packed. We were up to four to five hours to even see a doctor, unless you were actually very sick, of course. There were no available chairs.

People were even standing outside, patiently waiting to be triaged. It was a bit after midnight.

In walks 24-year-old "Gilligan" with his girlfriend in tow. I renamed this human after the lead character on **Gilligan's Island** circa 1964-1967. Watch one episode and you will better understand the following story.

Gilligan had been waiting for three hours to be triaged. This is about how it went:

Me: "Hi Gilligan. What can I do for you this lovely evening?"

Gilligan: "Well, I drove up to the mountains today and my ears popped."

Me: Pause. Pause. Pause. I began to look for the hidden camera under my desk, believing that I was being punked or being secretly filmed for an episode of **America's Funniest Videos**. Ok. I couldn't find a camera, so I began my line of questioning:

Me: "Do your ears hurt now?"

Gilligan: "Nope."

Me: "Are your ears popping now?"

Gilligan: "No."

Me: "Is there any drainage coming from your ears?"

Gilligan: "No."

Me: "So no blood or clear liquid is coming out of your ears?"

Gilligan: "No."

Me: "Are your ears painful to touch?" (I examined his ears.)

Gilligan: Touching his ears while stating "Nope."

Me: "Is that it?"

Gilligan: "Uh no. When we drove down the mountain, they popped again."

Me: Signing. "Of course. Ok Gilligan. I will have you go back out to the waiting room and a doctor will see you when they can."

Gilligan: "Is it going to be a long wait to see a doctor?"

Me: "Well Gilligan, did you happen to notice the large crowd standing around in the waiting room and outside and the 10 ambulances lined up at the ER entrance? It's probably going to be awhile."

Gilligan: "Uh, yeah. Does that mean it is going to be hours? Do I have time to go down the street and get some tacos?"

Me: "Gilligan, you probably have time to go to Mexico and get tacos. Just kidding." (I was NOT kidding.) But if you leave, we have to start over again and re-triage you. I suggest that you stay here in the ER."

Bottom line: May I suggest that a primary doctor would love to see patients with popping ears? I surmise that popping ears are also gladly seen by a doctor in an urgent care clinic. That is a much better use of medical resources. Again, the ER is severely impacted by such cases.

ER: Probably not the right address. But, due to laws, Gilligan was seen by an ER doctor and sent home at dawn.

With the huge growth in population, one would think it would be easy to identify the need for more healthcare facilities (i.e., more hospitals, and more clinics). How hard is that idea to figure out? The population is growing, for gosh sakes. People are flooding into the United States. All you have to do is walk into a hospital and look around for a place to sit. Head to the ER at 4:00-5:00 P.M. on any given day. The wait times are ridiculous.

Or better yet, watch them clear hundreds and hundreds of acres for a new planned housing community. Did anyone research, obtain statical data, or bother to use common sense? These humans will, at some point in their lives, need healthcare. Where will they go?

What the heck are planning committees, (Don't get me started on committees), along with hospitals, state and local healthcare administrators, and state and local governments, doing? Is there no foresight? Who the heck is not doing their job? Identify yourself, immediately! We need to talk.

I could've told you fifteen years ago that we would need more hospital facilities in my community. I worked in one. I lived in the trenches. I watched the increase in patient volume. Am I the only one who noticed?

Is the healthcare system and the government waiting for my approval? If so, go ahead and build the hundreds of hospitals that will be needed within the next 20 years. You have my approval.

OK, I may have exaggerated just a little. How about we start with two to three new ones in every large city.

Apparently, no one is noticing that A+B=C. (Yeah, for algebra!)

Suggestion:

Long patient wait times + more and more humans on this planet=Build more healthcare facilities…please.

Moving right along:

I got out of college in the early 1980s. Being a nurse was wonderful. We had plenty of supplies. We were expected to provide excellent care, 100% of the time to 100% of our patients.

We had the time and management support to care for your family like they were our own family members. We dressed, acted, and looked professional. Morale was up.

Florence Nightingale would have been proud.

What the heck has happened?

My opinion: For starters, we lost our "white!" We lost our professional look and attitude. Those of us who had the privilege of wearing white uniforms and a nursing cap from our university, with our name tags shining on our chest, our stethoscope around our neck, and our hair groomed up off of our shoulders, felt wonderful. Patients knew exactly who the nurses and doctors were.

As a bonus, we could bleach the hell out of the uniforms and thereby not only keep them white, but also destroy the yuck that was attached to them. We were "the shit!" We looked it, acted the part, and felt it.

We had worked so very hard to get our degree. We definitely wanted to represent our profession proudly, in dress and attitude.

I have felt saddened, annoyed, and embarrassed for our profession, many times during the last few years that I worked. Here is why:

Some healthcare workers, namely nurses, would arrive at the job wearing low cut t-shirts with business logos, tight pants, and make-up worthy of a magazine cover. Their hair would be flopping all over the place. Several of them didn't even look like nurses. They dressed like they were headed to the mall.

To make matters worse, many staff members spent most of their day, staring at their cell phones. Boy, oh boy. Values have changed over the past 10 years or so.

Suggestion:

If this describes you, listen up. If you are part of the **majority** of healthcare professionals who take pride in how we look, behave, and conduct business, well then help me convince your peers that this topic is important to our profession.

Dressing and practicing appropriately and for success are concepts that have moved away from some members of the medical profession.

How would you feel if your airline pilot showed up with a hangover, in a ripped t-shirt and shorts? Would it be ok for your dentist to keep looking at his phone, dressed in jeans and tank top, while you were having a root canal? Am I making my point?

The last department that I worked in, actually sprung for navy blue uniforms with the hospital logo for the nurses. Do you think everyone took advantage of this? Do you think all nurses started upping their game of dressing for success and pride?

Nope. The t-shirts still won out with some of the population. Pathetic.

Spending time doing anything other than patient care, and feeling ok with it, confuses me. How do medical people justify getting paid as a healthcare professional (lab tech, x-ray tech, nurse, doctor) when they are doing what I call, minimum daily requirements? Spending hours on a phone with personal calls is NOT in the job description. I am certain of that.

No one in management would take on that issue for fear of a harassment charge, I surmise.

Suggestion:

I contend that if you want to be treated like a professional and respected as such, you need to look and act the part. May I offer up the idea that you will feel more like a professional in a lovely uniform, hair groomed, and supplies in tow? Your patients will definitely appreciate it. If you use your phone only during breaks, won't your patients get more attention, and thus get better care from you? One of my mantras is treat all patients like they are your mother, providing you love your mother.

In conclusion, I remain thankful that these abhorrent behaviors are still in the minority.

Enough said. As you can see, I am not only devoted to nursing, but I'm also very passionate about treating patients and everyone for that matter, the way you would want your family to be treated.

Now that I am done capping on my sisters and brothers, here is another issue that may possibly be contributing to the lack of enthusiasm and professionalism at work:

Morale is way down. Nurses are working with little help, more responsibility, fewer supplies, and less staff. We are punched, kicked, spit on, and yelled at. People are rotten. We should have combat pay added to our salaries (and so should flight attendants for that matter).

Morale boosters from management are rare. I have offered many suggestions and carried out many morale boosters myself at work.

The bottom line is that nurses just want to feel loved, supported, and appreciated. Why is that rarely happening these days?

Suggestion:

I made this suggestion to several administrators.

Before every shift, administration would come into the breakroom and spit out any news. Just like our TV news, most of it was not good. And so, I suggested that administration interject something good, kind, or happy at the end of each morning report. Let someone (i.e. a tech or a nurse) know they are appreciated for a job well done. That would start us all off on an upbeat note for the day.

Nurses and techs would have the opportunity to thank a coworker or share a good work story. The administration agreed to this suggestion. That lasted about 3 days. Then it went back to "NBC NEWS!"

Next topic:

The role of the primary nurse in the ER has drastically changed:

Working inside the hospital as a nurse, I was able to focus on quality patient care and not tasks. I could educate my patients on procedures, discuss their plan of care, help them with their activities of daily living, etc.

Every department did its job. Lab drew blood. Respiratory therapists did breathing treatments. Pharmacists mixed their meds. Etc.

Life in the ER, long ago, was the same. Departments did their job.

Time has drastically changed the ER nurse job description.

In the ER, where life and death are constantly on the table, nurses are expected to do the work of all other departments including lab, respiratory therapy, dietary, pharmacy, etc. Who voted on these changes? Not me. Listening to, educating, and spending quality time with our patients to fulfill their needs, is officially over. There is no time for anything other than tasks. "Get them in and out, ASAP." Result: Nurses are exhausted, and people are not getting the care that they deserve.

Suggestion:

I believe that managers and hospital administrators have become way too busy and removed from the trenches to see what is happening. I invited several managers to spend a day taking care of patients with me. I wanted them to see that their expectations were unrealistic, unsafe, and **unbelievable!** No one accepted my proposal. My guess: If you face the truth, you will have to do something about it.

One of the hospitals that I worked at, put a suggestion box in the break room in order to "improve the workplace." I wrote approximately 19 suggestions for improvements. They ranged from adding plastic silverware in our break room for the staff to use (morale booster), all the way to "Please replace the T.V.s that were unable to be fixed in patient rooms." Some of them were broken for more than a year. Not one suggestion was taken, or used. Frustrating, at the very least.

May I suggest that we go back to staff meetings? Can we call them forums? Can they address the issues of the "working class?" Can the administration share with us solutions to these issues instead of saying, "Ok, we will take care of that," yet nothing is ultimately done?

I brought forth a suggestion: Hire someone, like an undercover boss, to spend time with the workforce. They could compile actual data and thus help make sentinel changes from the research they completed. I believe that is exactly what needs to be done. Again, that suggestion was vetoed.

I am certain that you have wonderful suggestions to improve things in healthcare. The question is, is anyone listening?

Listening or not, here are just a few more of my suggestions for improving the world of medicine:

Let's talk about the shortage of healthcare workers including doctors, nurses, and techs in every department.

The Covid pandemic pushed many healthcare peeps out of the profession. It tipped us over the edge. I was there. I was part of it. I was frustrated over the lack of administrative support, few protective supplies, and poor staffing, to name just a few issues. For many reasons, nurses left their wonderful professions either voluntarily or by force. I could write 10 chapters on that topic, but it would get much more intense.

(I am devoting most of the rest of this book to a funny, silly and sarcastic read.)

We need more healthcare professionals. No one would argue that fact. How can we recruit more healthcare peeps, you ask?

Suggestion:

May I suggest that clinic and hospital staff receive pay which is comparable to what football players make? How is it possible on this planet, and especially in the U.S.A., that someone who can throw a ball gets paid much, much, more money than a person who can, and does, save lives?

I just read that a quarterback signed a five-year contract for $255 MILLION DOLLARS! Say what? I can't even fathom that much money in a lifetime or 10 lifetimes, for that matter.

Many athletes get paid more than heart and brain surgeons. Try to comprehend this. Specialized surgeons go to school for an eternity. Some of them remove a heart from one body and place it in another human being, saving a life. Yet, they get paid only a fraction of what a person in their 20s gets for throwing a ball accurately. Crazy. Yet again, I'm on the wrong planet.

I love to watch football. Those athletes are incredible. I am happy for them. I am thrilled that their salary is OUT OF THIS WORLD. I just believe that healthcare workers are not always paid what they deserve, whether it be in money, benefits, or even kudos. Certainly, a boost in pay and benefits would be a step in raising morale.

Another suggestion:

Why don't more hospitals offer to pay for the medical education of a perspective nurse or doctor if that student agrees to work for them for a said period.

That seems reasonable. I believe that some hospitals do just that, but on my planet, they all should.

I am just full of ideas.

My opinion, and the opinions of many others (by others, I mean my friends): is that the healthcare profession is presently in shambles. The pandemic infected the medical profession making it quite ill. From wait times, to staffing issues, to supply issues, we are in a critical situation.

Medicine has become a big business. The "not-for-profit" is really "for profit." Administrators now believe that they can do the job for less: less supplies, less equipment, fewer hospitals, less staff, and it still runs, and everything is good. But it really isn't.

So, how does this rant that I have composed relate to you? What should you do about it, you ask?

I am about to give you some insider info. These suggestions come from experience. They are my ideas only:

a. If you are going to have an emergency, plan it for between 5:00-8:00 A.M. The ER is less busy at these times, usually. You will send me a thank you note if you ever get to experience this. Plan all of your emergencies so that they happen in the morning. Emergencies seem to happen later in the day because people tend to sleep in. People realize that they have an emergency after they have had their breakfast and a good cup of coffee. And so, the morning hours have less traffic, usually.

b. The ER is not a family vacation location. The hospital is loaded with germs because it is housing way too many humans with germs. Those germs tend not to adhere only to that human. If those contagious humans cough, sneeze, or do not wash their hands, and then they touch their body parts and then they touch anything in the hospital, anyone there can get sick.

And soooo…. why bring your 12 family members into the ED or hospital? Why oh why must you insist on bringing your nine-month-old baby with you? Please don't. I am trying to protect you, your babies, and your other family members from a catastrophic illness. Stay away from the ER unless you absolutely need it. Please.

c. The ER should not be used as your Dr.'s office. There are wayyyyy too many people on this planet, and still, the ER can't turn anyone away. That would be a legal violation. We have to see the entire world, and we do. This is why I am extolling the need to build more facilities and get more humans to agree to a life of service, similar to Florence Nightingale.

You are in luck, though. Most ER's have a "rapid care" or "fast track" area where they "op to punt" any human who has a "minor issue." Please, understand. The ER is trying to care for humans who may not live to see tomorrow. We are busy caring for peeps who are having strokes and heart attacks and want to jump off a bridge or slit their wrists. Our days are spent medicating the population who claim to have 10 out of 10 abdominal pain while they eat potato chips, drink a Coke, and text on their phones.

d. Medical people and EMS human beings need your love and support. They work hard doing things you would never want to do, even if you were paid one million dollars. Advocate for them. Shower them with hugs and kisses. Buy them gifts. Stand by them in a rally. Boost their morale in any way you can. I contend that without the medical community including first responders, humanity would cease to exist.

e. Nurses: For several of you and you know who you are: You want to be respected as the greatest profession on earth? Well then act like it. Dress professionally. Talk professionally. Put your phone away and spend more time advocating for and caring for your patients. (Drop the microphone.)

f. Write letters/email your governor, congressman, senators and definitely the President. They need to know about your experiences dealing with the healthcare system. They need you to advocate for more hospitals, more clinics and definitely more staff in every facility. They need to hear about your frustrations when trying to get a simple doctor's appointment and ending up having to go to the ER to get seen; because, "There are no available appointments today"; or "Your doctor is on vacation"; or because "There are no available appointments for three weeks"; (or a plethora of other reasons). Not enough nurses, doctors and other healthcare professionals, are causing definite delays in your care? Write a letter. Complain. Speak up.

g. If you have an issue, including not being happy with the care you have received, then go up the hospital chain of command, starting with the charge nurse and working your way up to the unit manager. Let them know what happened, how you feel about it, and what they should do differently. They may ignore you or actually do something about it. Hopefully, it's the latter.

h. Neither the charge nurse nor the unit manager has the power to make sentinel changes in healthcare. If you have major concerns about your family's ability to access, use, feel comfortable with, or obtain excellent healthcare, call your news station and report your concerns. Be proactive. Don't just sit around and complain. Do something about it. That is how laws get changed.

My own mother wrote so many letters to express her opinions to the President, senators, etc. that I would joke that she had her own file cabinet in the White House. If she felt an injustice, she wrote a letter. She stood for kindness and fairness for everyone. She (and my father) taught me the skill of standing up for what is right, just, and true. And soooo, SPEAK UP! Healthcare won't ever change unless WE CHANGE IT.

Me: Exhale

And So, We Laugh

I can't speak for all of the healthcare community, but I can speak for myself and the wonderful nurses who I have worked with across the USA when I declare:

Dealing with humans in healthcare can be a hilarious comedy show!

Humans are funny. They cause nurses to laugh, which is really helpful in a career that can take us to our knees in sadness. Sometimes we laugh so hard, we pee our pants, cough uncontrollably, hold our stomachs in pain, or have to leave the room, or unit, to compose ourselves. Some of these moments I jotted down for this chapter, in particular. What foresight on my part, aaaaa?

On any given day, many things occur in the world of medicine that make nurses, at the very least, smile. It could be a diagnosis, a simple comment by anyone, a doctor's order, a reason why a person sought medical care, a funny event that happened within the hospital, etc. We chuckle, giggle, laugh out loud, or laugh to ourselves. We sincerely thank humanity for doing this for us. Otherwise, nurses would probably quickly change careers and get a job as a barista. Afterall, some of us love our four + cups of coffee every work day. It keeps us going and thinking clearly. That's my story, and I'm sticking to it.

Taking care of humanity is one thing that makes us feel good inside, but the sadness 24/7 can get to us. There is a delicate balance to comforting others in their final moments, and staying mentally stable to protect our soul from its own demise. Caring nurses struggle with this daily, I assure you.

I found this quote somewhere and I kept it close to me for years:

If you stop caring, you're jaded.

If you care too much, it will ruin you.

I still can't read that quote without tearing up.

Sick humans in the hospital require a huge amount of physical, emotional and psychological time and energy from the staff. What I mean by that is sick humans are physically, mentally, and psychologically exhausting. The nurses, doctors, techs and all of the ancillary staff, for that matter, work their booties off.

There is never down-time any more for any of us medical personnel. There is almost no relief in the eight or 12 or 16 hours of stress at our jobs.

And so, laughing is OUR best medicine. It helps us to keep going. It breaks the tension and the sadness that we experience. It gets our minds off of horrible stuff, if even for a second. It resets us and our souls. It is like turning your phone off, waiting a minute, and turning it back on.

Something funny + laughter=We can continue on with our day.

(Algebra, yet again.)

Examples:

We were performing CPR in a room with about 15 staff members present. This is way too many staff members in that room at once, but we medical people love to save a life, and so we all went in to help out. Afterall, "We are all in this war together."

All of a sudden, someone noticed that this 89-year-old female who weighed 89 pounds, had the most beautiful fake breasts everrrrr. Actually, we all noticed this, but this particular staff member (who shall remain anonymous) said something like, "I should let Huge Heffner know that Mrs. Bunny, (I renamed her), is here in case he is looking for a center-fold for the next issue."

Although, technically, an inappropriate comment, we all laughed. This statement, by the tech, who was actually performing the chest compressions, broke the tension and freed our souls for a second or five.

(If the patient heard us, I know that she would have smiled, for she saw how hard we were all working to bring her back to life.) And no…she didn't make it.

But I will never forget her.

Another one:

I was working on a post-op/trauma 57-bed unit in South Florida. The nurses' station was in the center with long hallways/rooms on either side. There were no available beds. The unit was full.

Several of the nurses were at the nurses' station charting. It was in the days of paper charting from hell. All of a sudden, a very, very foul smell wafted across the air.

We all wrinkled our noses simultaneously. I asked, "What the heck is that smell?" Without missing a beat, Nurse K. fell to the floor laughing. Then another nurse started laughing, uncontrollably. Before you knew it, the entire staff in the nurses' station was laughing, except for me. I was bewildered. I couldn't figure out what was so funny.

"What's going on?" I asked. Nurse K., while still hysterically laughing, pointed to a bedside commode in the hallway, against a wall.

Seated on that commode, was a very old man, emptying his bowels along with sound effects. His colon apparently had been blocked for the past year. That is my guess, anyway.

Here is what I surmised happened:

The housekeeper had obviously cleaned the commode, but had not dragged it to the "clean utility area." Mr. D. (for doodie) was taking a stroll down the hallway when he came upon a toilet. "Aha," he must have said. "Perfect. I need to go anyway." And so, he did! Boy oh boy, did he!

My duty, (not doodie…lol) as the charge nurse, was to go over and assess the problem. Someone had to do it:

Here is how it went:

Me: Trying not to breathe through my nose, "Hi Mr. D. Is there a reason why you are going to the bathroom in the hallway?"

Mr. D: "Is this a toilet?"

Me: "Yes, it is."

Mr. D: "So I am using the toilet. Would you rather I go on the floor or in bed?"

Me: "Nope."

Mr. D: "Well then, get me some toilet paper. Please."

Me: I gave him the toilet paper. Yes, he wiped himself right then and there. No one, other than us nurses, saw it, as the hallway was empty of human beings at that time.

I helped him back to bed. I then picked my staff up off the floor after their fits of laughter. I emptied the bedside commode that was full, and I mean full. Ewwwww. (See why laughter is important?) I had a conversation with the housekeeper. We both laughed. Finally, I sprayed the hell out of the fourth floor with our hospital's "stinky relief spray."

Note to self:

-Keep hallways clear. Definitely don't leave any commodes in the hallway or anywhere other than the patient's room, right next to their bed.

-Even poo can be funny to nurses.

-Keep that "stinky relief spray on hand at all times."

-Gosh, I love the elderly.

-Gosh, I love my staff.

Next:

I worked in a very busy inner-city ER. Gangs would simply drop their "members" with gunshot wounds off at the ambulance entrance and leave. Many homeless and poor people also sought care there.

I loved working at that facility for many reasons: The staff was great; I learned a lot in a short period of time; and those who showed up for care usually really needed it.

One day, a 50-ish-year-old woman arrived in one of my rooms, complaining of chest pain. She was, shall we say, a large lady, at six feet tall and about 280 pounds. She had dark black hair and dark eyes. I would have guessed that she was a police officer at some point, or worked as a prison guard. She had a commanding presence. (You work with humans long enough, you can guess their profession. Boy, was I wrong.)

This lady was quite unhappy, in general. She definitely did NOT want to be in the ER.

Let's call her BOSS.

I decided to lighten the mood with conversation.

This is close to what happened, as I was about to start her IV:

Me: "So, can you think of any reasons that would cause this chest pain? Did you lift something heavy? Did you fall or injure yourself?"

Boss: "No. I don't lift heavy things. I make others do that. And no, I didn't fall."

Me: (Not realizing the significance of her prior statement until later). "Do you smoke?"

Boss: "No, I don't."

Me: "Did you strain yourself in any way?"

Boss: "Look! I haven't done anything new. I do the same things day after day. This chest pain is new. That's it."

Me: "I don't mean to upset you. I am just trying to figure this out."

Boss: "Right. Sorry. This is just my demeanor."

Me: (Ready to insert the IV needle into Boss's left antecubital vein and attempting to lighten the conversation). "So, what do you do for a living?"

Boss: "I'm a DOMINATRIX."

Me: Try to keep a straight face after that declaration. I was caught completely off guard and said, "That's nice. Must be fun."

Me: Thinking to myself as my face turned bright red: I can't believe that I just said that.

Boss: "Well, it pays the bills anyway."

This is not the end of the story…

I was feeding her nitroglycerin for her chest pain, every five minutes, when a unit secretary peeked into the room and asked me if her husband could come in to see her.

I am not sure why, but I assumed that dominatrix women are not the marrying type. That was a wrong bias of mine, apparently. Obviously, I know very little about that profession.

"Sure," I said, chomping at the bit in anticipation.

In walked a replica of Don Knotts. (If you have no clue who this actor was, google him. He starred in one of my favorite kid movies: **The Incredible Mr. Limpet**. It was a Disney movie in the 1960s. I probably watched it more than 20 times. You will not be able to watch that movie now, without thinking of this story in my book. Go ahead. Watch it. It is a great movie for kids. To give you an idea, Don Knotts was about 5 feet 6 inches tall. He weighed approximately 140 pounds. He was the definition of a nerd.)

Ol' Don walked in the room, ran over to his wife's bedside, and hugged her tightly. Note to self: He hugged her. She did not hug him.

I gave him a chair to sit in. That didn't last long because Boss did what Boss apparently does best: She began to boss him.

She started sternly telling him what to do including, "Get out of here and go home and clean up the kitchen from last night."

In conclusion, I had met my first dominatrix, but at least she had a job and was contributing to society. Whatever floats your boat.

Next: Translating English to English:

The following are two stories that happened to an English nurse who I worked with. She has since retired but was an excellent nurse. We have remained good friends.

I warned her several times that she would be in a book written by none other than me. These two work stories, I experienced with her, were too funny to pass up.

The first tale is about an elderly man who needed help getting to the bathroom. English nurse and I went into the room to help him. We both knew that his gait was unsteady.

She explained to the patient what she was about to do. We sat the patient up at the side of the bed.

All of a sudden, Nurse England swung around and started walking out of the room while stating, "I will be right back. I need to get a frame."

Patient: "What the hell does she need a picture frame for."

Me: "Beats me. Maybe she is tired of these bare walls."

English nurse returned with a walker. Who knew?

Apparently, a Zimmer frame or Zimmer is the word for a walker in England. The patient and I just chuckled and nodded our heads.

Here are a few other phrases and their translations from American English to England English:

"I will be your nurse." = "I will be nursing you."

"I will wake you up." = "I will knock you up." See how English from England can cause a fight in any bar or anywhere for that matter?

Fanny Pack = A rude word for your hoo ha.

I need to interject here:

I have several people in my life who are from England. They all have British accents and use lingo from their country. After hanging around them for years, I am now officially bilingual.

-trunk vs boot

-walker vs frame

-biscuit vs cookie

-French fries vs chips

-suspenders vs braces

-drug store vs chemist's

-stove vs cooker

-pacifier vs dummy (one of my favorites)

-garbage can vs dustbin

-apartment vs flat

-truck vs lorry

…and the list goes on and on

Next English nurse story:

There were three emergency room beds separated only by thin curtains. There was a man in each bed. They were not critically ill.

An English nurse was caring for the gentleman in the first bed. I was taking care of the guys in the second and third beds.

The English nurse said to the patient in bed one, loud enough for me and all three patients to hear, "I will be right back to nurse you."

All three patients and I begin to lightly chuckle.

The patient in the second bed announced loudly, "Can I trade nurses?"

The patient in the first bed said, "Hell no."

The patient in the third bed stated, "I'm next."

…and so, I took that lovely British nurse aside and explained the American definition of "to nurse," which is to feed a baby via your breast. We both laughed. We talk about that event even now, many years later, and we still laugh.

Ignorant or Uneducated?

Either Way, Let's Laugh

It's not just me. Many people will tell you, that on a daily basis, they are confronted with ignorant humans doing stupid things. We find those people everywhere: in our personal lives and experiences, at our jobs, out and about, or the second we turn on the news. Life is filled with them. It is a disease in our society that is obviously spreading fast. Scary. Very scary! But, it's also very funny sometimes, as well.

Stupidity is not just seen in those who are uneducated or psychologically-challenged. It does not only exist in those humans who live in a sheltered environment or in poor places. Brilliant, wealthy people do stupid things as well. Dumb humans are scattered all over our society, and in the world for that matter.

Ignorance is obviously a pandemic that has spread to the government. Just watch the news. You will see educated people who are ignorant.

Not only the media, but our government with absolutely NO medical background, has decided that they are capable of dictating the fate of a real pandemic. WTH? How does that happen? I could write 10 chapters on this topic.

I thought we were a democracy. I thought medical people handled medical issues and the media actually reported facts while the government handled laws, and so on and so on. Maybe that was just in the 1960s and 1970s with Walter Cronkite and President Kennedy. In the words of my wonderful sister Debbie: "The world has turned upside down."

Ok. I got a bit off track. These are just my opinions again, like it or not. No need to write me a political letter. You are welcome to your own opinion.

Anyway…

People void of common sense exist in every job. But this is my book, and so I will confine this topic to ignorant humans who I've come in contact with at work; humans who are missing the taco on the combo platter:

-a few clowns short of a circus.

-the cheese slid off of their cracker.

-their elevator does not go all the way to the
 top.

-dumber than a box of tacks.

-ran out of thread on their sewing machine.

-their antenna is not picking up all the channels.

-their belt missed a few belt loops.

-there is no grain in their silo.

-their bag of marbles has a hole in it.

Got the picture?

The thing is, I saw lots of people on a daily basis, simply by being a nurse and working in a bunch of hospitals in different cities across this country. I saw all walks of life, all ages, all colors, all ethnicities, all with various morals and values. I took care of little humans, big ones, poor ones and rich ones. Some had years of formal education and others had none. I am very happy to report, after my 65 years of existence on this earth, that most people actually have a brain and do use it.

Many other humans, however, have a brain but they don't use it consistently. And some, obviously, have NO BRAIN AT ALL!

Ignorance or stupidity might just be an occasional occurrence for someone. Gosh, we all have had our moments. Or, a human being may live in confusion at all times, or bliss, depending on how you look at it.

I often said at work, "In my next life, I want to be really stupid and gorgeous. I want to live happily, not knowing a thing about anything. I will marry a very wealthy man, 30 years my senior. I will sit on my yacht, travel the world and drink lemon drops." BTW, I have already invited my friends.

Back to the book: The point is that uneducated, ignorant, or uniformed humans can be very, very funny, as long as "no one loses an eye."

So, this is where I begin to share with you just a few award-winning stories (as voted on solely by me) about humans doing dumb, ignorant, uninformed, or uneducated things…or all of the above.

Let's begin with this story. It occurred years ago.

A male patient who was very sick, came into the ER. The staff was having trouble drawing blood, as this patient was quite obese. I called the lab and asked if a tech could be sent to the emergency room "stat" in order to draw blood on a very critical patient in room 12.

A lab tech arrived quickly and he successfully obtained blood specimens. We shall name this lab tech Lloyd after Jim Carrey in **Dumb and Dumber**.

After one hour, the doctor asked me to call the lab, as no results had been posted or called to the doctor.

I swear that I am not making this up.

I called the lab and asked to speak to the lab tech, Lloyd.

Me: "Hi, Lloyd. This is Robin in the ER. Do you have the results of the lab work on Mr. S. in room 12? You know, the blood you drew one hour ago?"

Lloyd: "I drew it stat. You didn't tell me to RUN IT STAT."

Me: Stunned. Bewildered. I thought that it was possible that Lloyd was kidding. Nope. Lloyd was serious. "Run it. Run it now," I yelled.

Stupid human. Definitely not funny.

Next one:

A mother arrived in the ER with her two-year-old daughter. Let's call the mother Rose, after Betty White's character on **The Golden Girls**.

Rose stated that her daughter had had the flu and a fever for two days. I checked the rectal temperature of the child, and the child's temperature was over 103F.

After the doctor examined the baby, he asked Rose if she had given her baby any Tylenol. Rose stated no.

Rose declared that if her daughter's fever had come down with the Tylenol, we wouldn't believe that the child was sick. Rose decided to hold off giving medication until the hospital staff took her baby's temperature.

That warranted not only immediate Tylenol, but also "lots-o-education" and a Tylenol dosing handout.

Rose was young and obviously an uninformed mother.

Once upon a time, my brother proclaimed, "I know what to do with my kid because I am a father."

The response from my fighter pilot, intelligent, and street-smart, father:

"You definitely don't need brains to reproduce. You just need to take part A and insert it into part B. Being "a father" does not make you smart or an expert in child-rearing."

When you are done laughing, feel free to read the next tale:

This one really bothered me. Here is what I remember:

I was one of the triage nurses. A teenager with obvious flu symptoms sat down in the triage chair. Her expensively dressed, "botoxed", snooty mother stood next to her.

Me: "Hello, my name is Robin. I am the nurse who will be taking your information."

At that moment, the teen turned her head away from her mother and proceeded to cough all over me.

Me: Handing her a little tissue box and stating, "Please cover your mouth so that the germs don't land on me. I don't want to get sick."

Mother: In disgust, "Boy, you are rude. You work in a hospital ER. You should expect to get sick. Don't tell my child what to do."

Teen: Simultaneously, while mother was bitching at me, "I am so sorry."

Me: (I had a lot to say but opted to keep my job. I was young at the time. In my later years, I would have handled it quite differently.) I immediately sent the teen to the minor injury area after triage was completed. The ER was busy so that was the appropriate place to send her. (That's my legally correct answer.)

My personal nursing diagnosis: Ignorant, uneducated and rude mother who had a lovely teen with the flu who I'd just educated.

Next:

The moon must have shifted. Venus must have squared another planet. Something catastrophic occurred, because overnight, the ER became EVERYTHING TO EVERYONE, just like a mother is. Word must have spread that the ER would help any human being with any issue, even dumb ones.

It happened in an instant, or so it seemed.

Suddenly, there were gurneys in the hallway, near the bathrooms, and I am guessing, soon to be on the ceilings. This is the norm for the ERs of today.

The ER became a dental office, the dermatology office to have your "nee nee" removed (my word for a growth of some sort on your body), a place to see a psychiatrist for "feeling anxious over the past year," etc. "Why is everyone using the ER for everything," you ask? My opinion:

1. They can't get an appointment with their Dr. for weeks or months. (I can sympathize.)

2. They can't get an appointment with the "appropriate address" for more time than they are willing to wait, like one day.

3. They can't sleep because they are worried about their nee nee. (See my next story.)

4. They have had a toothache for two weeks, have no dentist, and therefore they want heroine or meth to relieve their pain. "Lots of Norco will do." Plus, they think that the ER doctors went to dental school.

5. The ER is "where I always go because I have no insurance" but I have enough $ for tattoos, piercings, the latest cell phone, street drugs, etc.

6. They are just stupid.

For more of my rant on the improper use of the ER, please go to the chapter entitled "What Is Going on with Health Care."

I better stop here, or this topic will take up my entire book, and you will be writing me volumes of letters on "tolerance."

Next Story:

It was 2:00AM. I was the only triage nurse. I had one more hour of my 12-hour shift. It had been a really busy night.

A 27-year-old guy sat down in the triage chair. He was holding his arm like it was broken.

Me: Hello. How can I help you?

Him: He slapped his hand on the desk and pointed to a dot of discoloration. The dot on top of his hand was brown, and as small as the head of a straight pin. "Is this cancer?" he asked.

Me: Looking around for the "candid camera," thinking I was being filmed. "What makes you think that the dot on your hand is cancer?" I asked.

Him: "I watched the news tonight, and the news anchor said that a discoloration on your skin could be cancer, so I thought I would just come by the ER and get it checked out."

Me: Now my mind began reeling: Does this guy live alone? It is 2:00AM. Is he bored? Does he have any hobbies? (FYI: Hobbies are my cure for any illness, especially psych issues, which everyone has.) Was having sex not an option? (Sorry, it did cross my mind. He was an attractive engineer.) Why is he not sleeping?

My conclusion: This patient is intelligent, educated, yet stupid. He definitely made my book.

"Ok," I say. "Please have a seat in the waiting room, and the doctor will see you ASAP."

Yes, he waited and was seen by an ER doctor, who sent him home with a diagnosis of: "No cancer for you!"

The influx of complaints that are NOT emergencies is why we have standing-room only in the waiting room with waiting patients extending to the outside parking lot.

This is one of the 546,78 reasons (just my estimate; probably more than that) why the medical staff gets jaded and frustrated.

And thus, I definitely prefer socializing with my dogs, cats, birds, and even my chicken over human contact these days.

Drop the microphone.

Fortyish-year-old, well-dressed female, with fake everything, dragged her ten-year-old son into the ER.

Let me set the scene. This is very close to how it went:

It was noon and the ER was "busting at the seams." There were no available beds unless the patient truly needed emergent care.

I was, yet again, the only triage nurse for the day. It sure felt like all the funny stuff happened in triage.

Ten-year-old "Skip" (I will name him that for obvious reasons) comes hopping, and I mean skipping and hopping into my triage area. He sits in the chair. Mom was talking on the phone, obviously not really interested in me--or her child--for that matter. Let's call this mother Moira Rose, from the TV show **Schitt's Creek**.

Me: "Hi Skip. Can you tell me why you came to the emergency room today?"

Skip: "I don't know. My mom drags me everywhere." (from the mouth of babes).

Me: I looked at Moira Rose who was still talking on the phone. She pointed to Skip's legs and mouthed to me that she needed "a few more minutes" of this obviously unimportant phone call.

Me: "Do your legs hurt, Skip?" (He had now decided to leap out of the chair and jump around the triage room.) I said under my breath, but loud enough for his mother to hear, "Apparently not."

Moira: Covered the phone with one of her hands and said, "He was jumping off a curb and fell onto one of his legs. I don't know which one. I forgot. I want him checked out." She then went back to her phone call, laughing and chatting away.

Me: I instructed Skip to please come back to the chair so that I could assess him. Skip skipped and hopped over to the chair and sat down. I said, "Which leg is hurting you, Skip?"

Skip: Yelling at me, "NONE OF THEM! I told my mother that I was fine, but she hasn't gotten off the phone." (Smart kid.)

Me: I assessed Skip's legs and then I said, "Excuse me," to Moira. "Can we please talk?"

Moira: To someone on the other end of the phone: "I am so sorry but I will have to call you back. I am in the emergency room with my son who is in terrible pain with an injured leg. Talk soon." She then hung up the phone.

Me: "I can't seem to find any obvious deformities or abnormalities with either of Skip's legs. He is denying any pain and has been leaping and skipping around the room. Is there any other info you can provide to me? I will be happy to have him seen by a Dr. when one is available."

Moira: Without missing a beat, "How long is this going to take? I have a nail appointment in 45 minutes, and I can't miss it."

Me: "Not sure how long the wait is. We see the most critical patients…"

I could barely get out those last three words when Moira stated, "I guess you didn't understand me. I CAN'T miss this nail appointment."

Me: "Oh, ok. Now I understand. Have a seat in the waiting room and when a room is available, we will call you and your son in. A doctor will definitely examine him."

Moira grabbed her son by the arm and dragged him out of the triage area and out of the ER as he was yelling at her to "Let go of me." He was, of course, skipping. She was dialing her phone with the other hand, and heading out to get those nails done. I am sure of that.

As I sat back down ready for the next patient, I was hopeful that little Skip had a nanny to raise him.

And yes, for you triage police, we did follow up and call Moira to see if little Skippy was ok. And yes, he was just fine.

The mother had multiple diagnoses: Selfish. Uncaring. Doesn't Listen. And of course, Ignorant.

Skip was skippy. Sorry. I couldn't resist.

Next:

Should you know what the word "allergy" means by age 48 and married with three kids? Should you know what to do for a mild as well as a severe allergic reaction? Do you watch the news? Do you read anything? Are you alive, for gosh sakes?

I learned not to assume that humans have any sort of medical knowledge at any age.

In my opinion, every high school student in this country should be required to take a first aid class that includes CPR. This could be the difference between life and death with members of their family or friends. Educators could also use that class to drill into the heads of the youth, the absolute dangers of drugs, particularly street ones, that are killing kids these days.

I had to put that bit on educating our youth about healthcare issues somewhere in this book. Thanks for listening.

Case in point:

A forty-eight-year-old female came to the ER with c/o a light rash all over her arms, legs, and stomach that had started "two hours ago." No other complaints were offered and she was in no distress. The doctor questioned her regarding any allergies, contact with new products, etc. The patient vehemently denied allergies. The doctor ordered medication and left the room.

She started talking about her day, which included meeting her friends a few hours ago, for lunch. She followed this with, "Ooooo. I was told that I was allergic to shrimp a few years ago, but I thought that allergies just go away over time. I didn't really eat plain shrimp anyway. I had a shrimp salad instead. It can't be that, right?"

Me: No words. I needed a moment. I told her I would talk to the doctor. After speaking with the doctor, I returned to explain to her that shrimp is shrimp in any form. I told her that some allergies may disappear over time, like milk allergies, but peanut and shellfish allergies tend to be lifelong.

More education was provided.

And, I am definitely on the wrong planet.

I once read (don't remember where or when), that many adults operate, on average, at a third-grade level.

That seems about right.

Onward:

Sometimes, what we think is an ignorant human, is really just someone who is too young and naive to know better. I have always given young peeps the benefit of the doubt. Perhaps they have not had the education or information given to them. I don't classify those humans into the stupid category because they have not really lived on the earth for long.

According to me, once you have passed the age of 30 (give or take a decade), you should know stuff. Common sense should kick in. Before that, all bets are off, so I don't assume that young students or new graduates, who I train, know anything.

I have trained plenty of healthscare personnel in their 20s. I cut them plenty of slack. They are learning. They don't know stuff. They have but a few life experiences. They are somewhat uneducated, so I try to fix that.

I teach them how to be superior nurses because, after all, they will be taking care of me any day now.

And so here is a story about a young, newly-graduated male nurse who I trained.

We still laugh about it to this day.

Let's call him Joey, like the character on the TV show **Friends**. Got the picture?

Twentyish year-old Joey, had just graduated from college and had obtained his RN. He had been hired into the new grad program for the ER. He would be working alongside me for the next several months.

Joey needed to put a urinary catheter into this 80+ year-old, very confused female in order to obtain a urine sample. As his mentor, I was there to help.

I had him first gather the supplies and meet me in the patient's room.

There were three rooms in a row, separated only by curtains. The rooms were located right in front of the nurse's station. As I've already mentioned, curtains really don't provide much privacy in a hospital setting or anywhere for that matter. Everyone around us could definitely hear what was being said.

Note to self: Better let managers and administrators know this. Curtains don't provide privacy. They are apparently unaware of that fact.

I checked over the supplies that Joey had gathered. Perfect. They were all there. "Ok.

Go ahead," I said to Joey.

I watched Joey look at the catheter kit box like he was about to disarm a bomb.

"Go ahead," I repeated. Open the box."

It felt like it took him 30 minutes to unwrap that package. I literally clamped my lips shut so tightly that they hurt, so as not to say, "Move it; hurry up; it's not a bomb." I think I actually told him to go a bit faster on minute number five of that box opening ceremony.

Ok. The box was open. He was gloved. I went over the next steps with him. He nodded that he understood.

Now it was time to look at the target and clean it.

I positioned the patient and spread her legs open for Joey to see what he needed to see. I placed a blanket in a tent fashion over the patient's knees, which were bent, to give this poor, elderly, confused woman a bit of privacy.

More time went by. More encouraging words spilled out of my mouth. A review of exactly what he needed to do, was completed by me, verbally. Still nothing happened. More pleas to begin the procedure. Still nothing.

"Let's go," I said gently. "You can do this." He was just staring at this very old woman's HOO-HA. (my word for a woman's private part south of the equator).

"Just do it," I finally said in a kind but very firm voice.

All of a sudden, Joey started poking the catheter very, very gently, all over the woman's hoo-ha.

"What are you doing?" I yelled. He immediately stopped what he was doing and stated, "I don't have much experience down there." Joey stepped back and put the catheter back on the tray.

This event was immediately followed by loud laughter from the other two patients (separated by the curtains) and hysterical laughter from the staff at the nurse's station.

I had nothing to say other than, "You just made my book."

I took over the procedure and explained to Joey, as he watched intently, everything that I was doing.

When the catheter was in, the patient was comfortable and tucked in bed, and the audience had quieted down, we both walked out from behind the curtain.

Standing there was a doctor. He simply put his arm around Joey's shoulder and guided him into the doctor's office, saying, "Come with me Joey. I am about to give you a talk on the "birds and the bees."

Joey was NOT stupid. He was just uneducated.

FYI: Joey grew up to be a charge nurse in the ER and now works on a trauma helicopter, saving lives. Proud teacher here.

Last story in this chapter: This patient's response felt initially stupid, but now sounds intriguing. (kidding)

Forty-five-year-old man with urinary issues:

Me: "Now that I have removed your urinary catheter, I am giving you this urinal so that I can measure your pee pee."

Patient: (with a straight face and with sincerity) "You don't have to measure it. I know it is exactly 6" soft.

Me: Stunned. Speechless.

My thoughts:

-I obviously should have said "to measure your urine" instead of pee pee. A valuable lesson. Pee pee could mean peeeeeeeee **or** your penis.

-Why was he measuring his DICK, soft? Is that something men do often? Is that a normal activity to complete yearly, for a 45-year-old male? Note to self: I will ask my brother.

Does he have any other hobbies? (I swear that hobbies cure everything.)

Was he stupid? Just a funny misunderstanding, I hope.

We will leave it at that….

Robin's Believe It or Not

I remember as a child; I'd watch a show about funny things kids say. A man would interview children. They would answer his questions with sincere honesty. The kids were also quite animated while they answered his questions, and so the interview was usually very funny. **Kids Say the Darndest Things.**

Well, let me break it to you: Humans, of all ages, say and do funny things. I know this to be true. I have worked with the public for 40 years. Shall we include my other jobs prior to nursing? If so, add another 10 years to that figure.

The word "funny" is a broad term. Events and things that I consider funny, may be considered dumb, silly, stupid, odd, weird, unusual, embarrassing, crazy, or offensive by others. Do you get the picture? Humor is subjective.

And so, I will reminisce and share with you, in this chapter, some admissions to the hospital and ER stories that made me laugh, or at least smile. I only hope you experience the same reaction.

I spent over ¼ of my career working on various units inside the walls of a hospital. Simply put, a patient needed doctor's orders to receive care. An admitting doctor would compose pages and pages of orders for those patients who actually had a valid reason for being right where they were. Even so, some of the reasons that were recorded for admission to the hospital, were very funny.

Emergency room patients come under a completely different heading. Frequently, the odd ones appear suddenly and knock you off balance. They show up like Dracula in the London fog.

For example, my work day in the ER was passing by uneventfully, peacefully, and quite lovely, when all of a sudden, a man in his early 40s, as I recall, was placed in my assigned area. I went into the room for the purpose of assessing him and finding out why he decided to come visit me.

We shall name him American Senior Sniper or Ass, for short.

Mr. Ass was pacing inside of the room while holding his rear end with one hand. He refused to get onto the gurney. He did agree to change into a hospital gown.

Mr. Ass told me, with all seriousness, that he was camping, when suddenly he slipped and fell backwards in his tent, onto three small, plastic, green, army men. They were now located "pretty high up" his butt and he needed them removed ASAP. "Please. They hurt terribly," Mr. Ass stated.

Try to get that visual out of your head. This story is permanently branded in my brain.

I recalled seeing my brother launch those army men around the yard, when we were kids. I knew that those green guys held rifles and swords. Ouch. I felt Mr. Ass's pain.

I notified the doctor that her next patient was in quite a bit of discomfort. I relayed his story to her.

I chose to let the ER doctor give him an anatomy lesson and explain why plastic anything does NOT simply jet up one's bootie "accidentally." Don't you worry. This lovely female ER doctor could be heard down the hallway giving him an extensive lecture.

I have plenty of bootie stories, as most nurses do. I will only share a few more in this chapter. Not interested? You are free to skip them and head to the next chapter. Caution though: "Rear end" stories are scattered all over this book, plus these stories are really funny.

Next story:

I received a female, pre-op patient. I had to get her ready for surgery. I was a young traveling nurse at the time, working on a pre-post op surgical unit. I was very naïve.

The diagnosis on the admitting paperwork read, "Foreign Object." I don't remember the rest of the diagnosis, but that UFO was somewhere, lost in space, and required a surgical colon resection.

Apparently, husband and wife were having a "rough sex" evening after consumption of a large amount of alcohol. Mr. Husband decided to shove a vibrator, in the on position, up into Mrs. Wife's bootie, as far as he could, to where the "sun don't shine." Weeeeeeee!

After an x-ray, it was determined that their toy made its way to Pluto, and thus surgery was in order.

Furthermore, that sex toy was still vibrating and the patient could feel it. She insisted that I put my hand "here" on her abdomen, so that I could feel the vibration. I did what she wanted me to do. I was a "deer in headlights" as I palpated her abdomen and felt the vibration.

That whole encounter scarred me for life.

She was taken to surgery immediately and eventually discharged home without any further incident, and hopefully with post-op info on how to use that thing correctly.

Last bootie story in this chapter. One of my favorites.

It was a busy day in the ER, as usual. I walked into room 30 to meet my new patient. He looked exactly like Santa Clause. He was tall with white hair, a long white beard, and a very round belly. I could visualize children sitting on his lap and sharing their Christmas toy lists with him.

This is what I remember to be true:

Me: "Hello. My name is Robin. I am your nurse. I get to take care of you today. Can you tell me what I can do for you?"

Santa: "Yah. Get the dildo out of my ass. It is starting to hurt, and I can't get it out."

Me: Blank stare at him. I was stunned. I was shocked. Aren't you shocked as well? My emotions then switched to sadness. He destroyed my view of Santa Claus. Santa would NEVER do such a thing.

"I will be right back. I am going to speak with your doctor," I said.

It gets better.

I meandered into the doctor's office area. I started to discuss this patient with the senior physician who was assigned to Santa, but this doctor cut me off and told me to "speak to him," as he pointed to a young doctor, who looked about 16 years old.

This was the first day on the job for young Dr. Green.

I am naming him Dr. Green because he had just finished his residency and this was literally his first day out of school. Fortunately, he was being precepted by a funny, crusty, old ER doctor.

I reviewed Santa's complaint with Dr. Green. He listened. He looked confused and terrified. Dr. Crusty, our wonderful ED, seasoned doctor, heard the rundown and noted the "puppy's" confusion. He offered up the following suggestion that went something like this: "Just glove up, use lots of lube, and pull that sucker out."

Dr. Green still looked frightened to death but said, "OK."

I left the doctor's office to greet my next patient who had just arrived in the room next to Santa.

Apparently, the nurse who was in charge of that area of the ER, assisted Dr. Green in removing the sex toy from Santa's rectum. Unbeknownst to me, the nurse placed that XXL dildo in a bedpan. She placed that bedpan in the garbage container in the room, on top of the existing garbage, that was filled to the brim. The lid barely closed shut.

This is where the story gets really good.

Santa left; the toy stayed.

The next patient arrived in the same room. She was an 80ish year-old woman with chest pain. We shall rename this patient Estelle, after Estelle Getty from **The Golden Girls**. She looked the part.

Estelle's husband sat down in the seat, drum roll please, located right next to that garbage can.

I was unaware that the last patient's toy had a new home: just under the lid of the garbage, right next to Estelle's husband.

Mr. Husband lifted the lid of the garbage can to throw out a tissue. The baseball bat looking dildo, freshly removed from the prior patient's bootie, was lying gently in a bedpan, on the top of the rest of the garbage.

Mr. Husband stared at the used toy, which was at his eye level. He looked bewildered and confused, as he stared at the UFO, while holding the garbage can lid up.

I was busy placing Estelle on the heart monitor and blood pressure cuff. Glancing over at Mr. Husband, and due to my fine-tuned assessment skills, may I add, I dropped the blood pressure cuff onto the bed. I flew through the air in .01 of a second and slammed the garbage lid shut, luckily avoiding damage to Mr. Husband's hand. I then apologized and dragged the trash can into the hallway. I immediately paged overhead: "Housekeeping stat to the hallway in front of room 30, for trash removal."

Yes. That was a teachable moment for the helper nurse and Dr. Green. Never, ever leave sex toys in a patient's room. We all laughed.

Yes, I did apologize to Mr. Husband, for an overfilled garbage can. I ignored discussing with him, the elephant in the room, rather the XXL dildo in the garbage. I'm sure that he had no idea what it was. At least, that is my story and I'm sticking to it.

As the dildo was being transported to the incinerator, I declared, "This made my book." And it did.

Off of the "foreign objects vs butt" stories now:

Once upon a time ago, I worked on a med-surg unit in a community hospital. Across the street was a facility for the criminally insane. Yes, CRIMINALLY CRAZY! These humans did terrible things to other humans: **Silence of the Lambs** stuff. "Lose sleep over never even knowing what they did" kind of stuff.

Anyway, if any of these Jeffrey Dahmer kind-o-people had medical issues, these problems were fixed on the unit where I worked.

Those were the patients who I cared for, for one year, until I had had enough.

Picture this: My first contact with one of these so-called humans:

Here I was, just out of nursing school, in an all-white uniform with a nurse's cap. I was completely innocent and naïve. I went sauntering into the room where a "Jack the Ripper" sort of character was chained to the bed, accompanied by two police officers with guns.

Smiling, I said, "I have your medication for you, Jack."

The patient smiling, with the look of a serial killer, attempted to leap out of bed, stopped only by truck towing chains attached to both limbs and around his waist. They were secured to the metal frame of the bed. The bed weighed as much as a small car, thank God.

Next story:

On a particular day, I was asked to help with a GI procedure on one of those lovely crazies. A teenage girl, who had done harm to her family, as I recall, was now housed across the street. She was obviously very hungry or very upset because she had swallowed a ton of jewelry. I don't remember where she got it from. X-rays confirmed that her stomach was a gold mine, literally.

An experienced GI nurse was sent to assist the GI doctor with the endoscopy. I was just there as a backup or runner if the two of them needed anything. That was a good thing, because at that time, I had never assisted with a GI procedure.

I stood in the room, not moving, as the procedure began. I was afraid of this girl patient. She had a permanent "Chucky doll" grin. She looked very scary. I remained hopeful that the chains around the patient + the two police officers present, would equal protection for me from this psych patient.

The GI doctor was a little scrappy guy and the GI nurse looked way too nice to assist with any mayhem. My heart was beating out of my chest.

Anyway, the procedure began, the teen went into a twilight sleep, and so I relaxed a bit.

The Dr. started pulling gold chains and charms out of this girl's gut. I felt myself getting nauseated. I was about to throw up when the Dr. stated, "If this next one's a Rolex, I get to keep it."

Uncontrollable laughter filled the room. My nausea subsided. No Rolex was excavated. The patient recovered and was sent back across the street.

Out of the criminally-insane stories and on to the ER tales:

I was taking care of a man in his 80s. Let's call him Kramer, as in Jerry Seinfeld's sidekick. Kramer came in with chest pressure that had started a few hours before his visit to the ER. He had a history of angina.

I was reviewing Kramer's medication list with him, calling out each drug on the list, and asking him if he still took the named med. I noted that he was on Viagra, a potent vasodilator that treats high blood pressure as well as erectile dysfunction. I was about to give Kramer nitroglycerin, another potent vasodilator for his chest pain. I had to ask Kramer if he had taken Viagra in the last 24 hours, as Viagra + Nitroglycerin=potential for a sharp drop in blood pressure.

The conversation went as follows:

Me: "Kramer, I need to review your medication list with you. Please let me know if you take these medications."

Kramer: "Ok."

Me: "I see that you are taking Viagra. Did you take any in the past 24 hours?"

Kramer: "No," he said with a smile on his face. "Am I going to need some?" he asked and then winked at me. "One can hope," he stated.

We both laughed.

Another story about an elderly man:

I was taking care of a 90-year-old man who was alert and oriented. We shall call him Kev from Ricky Gervais's Netflix series, **Derek**. If you haven't watched this brilliant series, you are missing out. It is not only hysterically funny and completely inappropriate, but it's poignant and heartfelt at the same time. In the show **Derek**, Kev is a highly-sexual alcoholic.

Anyway, I was attaching the monitor leads to Kev's chest. I reached over him to place a lead on his left chest when I felt a hand encompass my left breast.

I looked down to find Kev holding my breast. I quickly removed his hand and sternly stated, "Why did you just grab my breast?"

Kev smiled and said, "Because I can. I am 90 years old. I have nothing to lose!" We both laughed.

The Lab

No matter what hospital I have worked in…

No matter what unit I have worked on…

It is the same story over and over again.

The nemesis.

The Darth Vader.

The thorn in any nurse's side.

Them vs Us.

Who am I talking about? **The Laboratory**.

They have the control. We never win!

It's a love-hate relationship.

Let's just start with this:

Why are your test results not back yet, or why is the lab taking so long to process the blood sample, you ask?

Here are some of the reasons why, per the lab staff:

"We didn't process the lab you sent because it was hemolyzed":

In medical terms, hemolyzed means that the red blood cells have broken open. It can happen if the needle that is used to draw the blood, is simply too small, or if the blood is wrongfully shaken up in that test tube, or it may be due to a plethora of causes that I intend to address below. The potassium that lives in the cell jumps out of the cell into the blood and can cause an elevated potassium reading.

Now, from a nurse's standpoint, get ready…I sound angry…and you would be too after torturing your patients over and over again to get blood, only to be told it wasn't any good.

Solutions, that I have formulated, to solve the hemolysis issues:

1. Weekends: Saturday and Sunday in particular. I am unclear if there are different staff members who complete the lab tests on weekends or if the moon changes on weekends, or if the war (ED nurses vs lab) begins on Saturday mornings and ends on Sunday nights. The fact remains that we nurses walk around all weekend, every weekend, shaking our heads and grumbling as we torture our patients over and over again for the purpose of redrawing their blood work, that was "hemolyzed." The quantity of calls from the lab increases on weekends. The story is always the same, only the patient's names are different: "The specimen you sent on Mr. Jones is hemolyzed," the lab tech states.

Hemolysis seems to occur many more times on weekends per me. Why is that?? No one seems to know.

In my opinion (and I have a lot of those), nurses have actually found a solution to this problem that makes us feel better:

"Let's be passive-aggressive." If the blood specimen is hemolyzed, we simply call the lab tech and say, "We are having trouble drawing blood. Can you please come draw the specimen?" Only then does collecting and processing blood seem to work without a hitch on weekends.

Call enough times for lab to come draw, and the quantity of hemolysis plummets. Don't believe me? Ask a few ED nurses.

Next:

2. Improper tube mixing: We send all blood tubes and lab work to the lab via a tube system. That tube system travels at 30 miles an hour, per my guess.

Don't get excited because that tube system is frequently broken and so, we nurses or techs have to walk the lab tubes to the lab. (Just add that to the other jobs that we do in one shift.)

Did any genius architect consult a nurse or lab tech to see if any "shaking of the blood tubes" occurs enroute inside of a tube system? The route to the lab via a tube, is the same distance from the entrance of Costco to the toilet paper location. The lab tubes are being jet-propelled through the walls of a hospital.

Does it seem feasible that violent shaking could break open blood cells? Is common sense as scarce as low food prices these days?

In actuality, some tubes need to be shaken and some not. Maybe we need to notify the tube system which tubes are ok to shake and which ones aren't. Crazy.

Onward:

3. Incorrect filling of tubes/excessive suction: our blood tubes have suction inside of them that simply suck the blood from the patient's arm. We have no control over how fast that happens. It just does it by magic.

Has no one in lab or management thought of this? THE TUBES FILL THEMSELVES. They "eat until they are full." Then they stop filling. If it is a suction problem, call the tube company. Yes, admittingly, nurses sometimes use a syringe to draw the blood, and that situation could possibly, not definitely, be our fault.

4. Incorrect needle size can cause hemolysis: We are in the EMERGENCY ROOM for gosh sakes. We like big needles. The big needles help us save lives by getting meds and blood into people faster. We only use baby needles if our patient's vein is smaller than a single hair. "We use the appropriate needle that fits the vein," I say, being politically-correct.

I often image that when a lab tech calls and says a specimen is hemolyzed, what they really mean to say is one of the following:

1. "I dropped the specimen, and it broke open all over the lab floor." Ewwww.

2. "I let it sit on the counter too long, and it is now one big clot."

3. "I forgot where I put that darn tube. It is in the lab somewhere."

4. "Oh. Is it in the drop-off box? I didn't look there."

Enough on hemolysis. Onto the real issues:

As a proactive nurse who knows that most lab specimens, which are sent from the ER, should be processed in under two hours, I often call a bit before the two-hour mark to see if I can retrieve the results, to ultimately help the patient get the heck out of the ER.

Other than hemolysis, here are a few of the other reasons, given by the lab techs as to why no lab results are available:

- "There is not enough blood in the tube." (You mean the tube that self-sucks? Did you notify the tube itself? When were you going to tell me?)

- "We did not receive the blood." (WTH? I sent it in that "reliable" tube system that was just updated and cost this hospital $785,647 to upgrade.)

- "The lab tech is at lunch and has not started testing the blood you sent." (Is there only one tech in this huge hospital?)

- "The other lab tech is on break." (Holy hell.)

- "The other lab tech is in the bathroom." (OK, that I understand.)

- "The machine is broken." (Again?)

- "This particular lab test has to be sent to a regional lab." (So, we won't have the result for days? Were you going to call me or the doctor and let us know this important information?)

- "The machine is being calibrated." (Whatever that means and entails…)

And my very favorite:

- "It is being run right now and will be posted when it is ready." (This probably means they appreciate me reminding them to run the lab.)

In conclusion, to "lab techs from hell" (no offense, lab techs):

Nurses have tons of other things to take care of with our very sick patients. I don't expect you to clean poop or shove tubes into human beings the size of garden hoses. So please come draw your own lab if you don't like what you get. After all, you are the lab tech.

There. I finally got that out, after 40 years of lab issues stewing in my gut. I feel better now.

The real truth…The honest to God real truth:

We actually love our lab peeps. ("Boy Robin, it doesn't sound like that.")

Right, but remember what I said: It's a love-hate relationship.

We really appreciate our lab peeps. They help us. When we are exhausted from trying to get blood out of a human potato, they show up and save us. We befriend them so they will help us. We beg for their help, promising them food from the break room. We tell them we love them, which we do. (I know I already said that, but I want them to be on our side.)

The lab techs are our heroes, especially in a critical situation when nurses are busy doing CPR, giving critical meds, putting tubes in every single open hole that a human has, mopping the floor of yuck so no one trips, etc. Ok, you get what I am trying to say.

99% of lab techs according to me, but definitely not fact-checked, are able to find a vein on a tile. Of course, "there is always one" lame tech who will show up on your bad day from hell and not be able to find a vein to draw from.

We DO need them.

We DO love them.

They are an essential part of healthcare.

ROCK ON LAB TECHS!

Ok. Because I need to end this section on a funny note, here is a true lab story that happened to me. It was so odd, that I knew that it would make my book.

Me: "Hello. ER. This is Robin. Can I help you?"

Lab: "Who is this please?"

Me: "This is Robin." (2nd time)

Lab: "How do you spell that?"

Me: "With an "i" like the bird."

Lab: "I would like to report a high potassium level."

Me: "OK. On who?"

Lab: "It doesn't matter. It was from two days ago. Someone redrew the lab at some point, and it was normal. I just need to report this and get a name to write down on this paper."

Me: "Huh? What? (To myself: WTF?)

Lab: "We had an abnormal lab value on Mrs. M. We didn't report it to ER. We should have. The lab was redrawn by someone and it was normal."

Me: "Yah. Soooo?"

Lab: "So I just need a name to put down on that report."

Me: Pause. "Ok. My name is Sylvia with a y!"

The Pharmacy

Some time ago, supermarket administrators decided that the population could, without any training, become grocery store clerks. The CEOs of stores forgot that some humans on this planet operate on a third-grade level.

On that note, I have surmised that the amount of free food leaving the grocery store, on any given day, due to operator error, equals the salary of one clerk. It's a wash.

I just recently learned that if you take the hand scanner, and scan the dime-size tag on fruits and veggies and plop them on the scale, you don't have to push the "search for item" button. I thanked the one clerk who showed me that little ditty and told her she had just given me my one and only orientation to my newly, unpaid job.

Why am I discussing grocery shopping and the punting of the check-out process, you ask? Similarly, someone in a hospital decided that nurses could be pharmacists and pharmacy techs with minimal formal training. This became job number 583 punted to registered nurses. (Approximately.)

Apparently, the same so-called-humans who think that the world population could check themselves out of a supermarket, also believe that the scant drug training that nurses received in school (for me it was four decades ago) was enough training to mix, know about, and give, all the drugs ever invented, CORRECTLY to patients. This includes the new ones that appear in our Pyxis, the drug dispensing machine, every other day.

Just for that reason, I vote that we add registered pharmacist to our badges.

Again, I am not going to speak for the entire planet. I will, however, speak about my experiences with The Pharmacy.

When I became a nurse, and for many years after that, pharmacists mixed almost all medications and sent them to us to give to our patients. Then, somewhere along the line, nurses were given the job of mixing certain medications including antibiotics and potassium. Potassium mixing was swiftly taken away from nurses, probably due to some sentinel event, I surmise. Did I have a class on how to mix and give every med, you ask?

Nope. If so, I don't recall those classes. Apparently, someone deemed classes in algebra and Florence, across her lifespan, much more important to my success in nursing.

Fortunately, on any given day, there are aways several nurses who know exactly how to deal with every issue that arises. Those super nurses are always very young, bright-eyed, and on overdrive. They have been my instructors on several occasions, in my later years, especially when new equipment or processes appear out of nowhere, without warning or education.

Thank goodness there are also drug books and computer pages that tell us how to mix meds; give them; their side effects; adverse reactions to watch out for, etc. Those books are essential to a nurse's survival and yours as well.

In order to mix any IV medication that will be given in drip form, there is a "chee chee" to attach. (See definition of a chee chee in the chapter entitled My Mantras and My Words.) One end of the chee chee is placed in the vial of medication, and the other end of that chee chee goes into the bottom port of the IV bag. I have probably experienced five to seven new and different chee chees without any formal education. They just appear in the med room, by magic. They all require a different way of attachment. After years of fighting with those devices and finally recruiting the help of much younger, super nurses, I am now an experienced chee chee operator. But, should I, your nurse, be spending time trying to figure out that kind of stuff? Shouldn't mixing meds be a pharmacy job? Just saying.

On my planet, mixing medications is the sole responsibility of the pharmacist. End of.

Here is a shout out to pharmacists. We definitely need them.

Thank goodness, a pharmacist is only a phone call away. When I am finally off "hold" and transferred to an actual pharmacist, I feel like I am on the phone with a saint. They are knowledgeable human beings who are able to answer all my questions, including:

Does this med need a filter, and if so, what kind?

This is a new med. (I have already looked it up in **The Nursing Drug Book**) Is there anything that I should be especially aware of? Etc. Etc.

I really do appreciate the vast knowledge that a pharmacist has. Because constant changes occur in the world of drugs, there is no way that any nurse could keep up with these modifications.

Next topic: Getting a medication from pharmacy=Seemingly impossible.

It is easier to buy a new car from a dealership. Easier to give birth, I surmise. Easier to have BRAIN SURGERY. Ok, ok. Maybe I went a bit too far. (If you are a nurse, you are probably yelling at me that I didn't go far enough.)

Case in point: I will "bet the farm" that the following situation has happened to many nurses if not all.

Let's just say a doctor orders a new medication for a patient in the ER. Also, let's say the doctor stated that he wants the patient to get that newly ordered medication as soon as I was able to get it from pharmacy. Let's also note that this ER is the size of a Costco and divided into four or five sections. The pharmacy is invariably located a mile away from the ER. Here is how a conversation with the pharmacy usually goes:

Me: "Hi pharmacy. I am still waiting for that medication Dr. House ordered an hour ago. Can you send it?"

Pharmacy tech: "Hold on. Let me check."

Minutes tick by.

Pharmacy tech: "Yes. We have that order."

Me: "Good. Can you please send it now?"

Pharmacy tech: "Sure can."

Another half hour goes by.

Calling the pharmacy again:

Me: "Hi pharmacy. Still waiting for the medication on Mr. Sickly that Dr. House ordered." (Made up names.)

Pharmacy tech: "Hold on. Let me check."

Minutes tick away.

Pharmacy tech: "Yes. We have that order."

Me: Deep breath: "I know you do. This is my second phone call for a medication. The doctor wants it given to the patient ASAP. Can you send it immediately?"

Pharmacy tech: "Sure. I will get it in the tube system as soon as the pharmacist checks it."

Me: "Thanks."

Another 20 minutes go by.

Me: "Helloooo! Pharmacy. Looking for the medication you were sending 20 minutes ago on Mr. Sickly who is really sick now. Did you send it?"

Pharmacy tech: "Hold on please."

(My blood pressure is rising fast.)

Minutes tick by.

More minutes tick by.

I hang up and call back:

Me: "Hello. Please don't put me on hold. Please tell me that in one second, I will receive the medication due long ago, for Mr. Sickly."

Pharmacy tech: "Hold on please."

Me: String of cuss words fly through my brain and I don't cuss…much.

Pharmacy tech: "The medication is located in the Pyxis in section one of the ER."

Me: To myself: WTF? Why didn't he tell me that an hour ago? "Pharmacy, I am in section 5. That is about a half mile away. (The distance from the entrance of Costco to the location of the laundry detergent.) Is there a reason you can't send it IMMEDIATELY to section 5 in the tube system?"

Pharmacy tech: "I just thought it would be faster if you went to get it there."

Me: "Apparently it is. May I suggest that the next time you get a medication order from the ER, and I call you several times regarding the location of that medication, you let us know where you are hiding it on phone call #1? Just a thought."

Pharmacy tech: "If you want me to send it, I can. I just have to find a pharmacist to check it."

Me: (I had already pulled out several hairs from my head) "Nope. I will go hike to section one, and leave my sick patients to fend for themselves for the 30 minutes it will take to pick up the medication. Have a nice day."

…and these are the people who are checking out their own groceries!

Psychiatric and Substance Abuse Patients

Are humans born crazy? How do people become crazy?

Most of us older folks came into this world with a clean slate. We were taught by our parents, teachers, TV personalities, friends, etc. how to behave and what was acceptable or unacceptable. Drilled into us over and over again, was the concept of right vs wrong. At least, that is how it was in the 1950s, 1960s and 1970s. That is how it was in my life. I'm not sure what happened after that.

Child rearing has always been trial by fire. Dr. Spock (NOT the Star Trek guy) wrote a simple, common-sense book for mothers on how to care for a sick child. It was a sort of Bible to new mothers. It certainly worked for my mother with four kids.

I was raised by an Air Force, fighter pilot, father (who came out of New Jersey) and a gentle, kind, yet firm mother. Lines were clearly drawn. "Behaving" was the ONLY option.

Humans in this country, in those days, were punished for amoral or unethical behaviors. That is how I remember it.

If we were bored, we were told to "find something to do" like play a sport or get a hobby. We played neighborhood football, kick the can, tag, etc. We would finger paint, string necklaces, or color in a coloring book. Getting into trouble was NOT an option.

We lived in a middle-class neighborhood. None of my neighbors had much money. It was up to us kids to find entertainment. And so, we did. We found things to do that didn't involve crime.

No, my childhood was not perfect, but due to the fact that discipline was enforced, good and evil were identified, and right vs wrong was clarified and dealt with, I think that I turned out pretty well.

Speed forward to now: Some kids and adults can choose to riot, steal, lie, and cheat with little punishment from inside the home, classroom, or from society in general. Antisocial behavior is "no big deal." You will be in and out of jail in seconds, if you end up going at all. My opinion.

Chaos. This planet has turned into a chaotic mess.

Apparently, child rearing has taken a hard left for some. It's like part of society has run amuck. Any behavior is acceptable, tolerated, or ignored until a sentinel event occurs, like a mass shooting. At that point, the parents notoriously say, "I had no idea." WTF? Your son is building weapons in your garage, and you had no idea? I am lost. I know what my dogs are doing at any given moment.

There has to be a reason that your kid's brain thought it would be ok to kill another human. Remember, they were born with a clean slate. Or were they?

Case in point:

This patient gave me nightmares for years. He still makes the hair on my neck and arms stand up when I think about him.

I was a triage nurse on this particular day. In walked a father and son. The son sat down in a chair, next to my desk. The father walked to the other side of me, which felt odd. Usually, families stand next to each other in the triage area.

This is pretty close to the what occurred:

Me: "Hello. My name is Robin. I am the triage nurse. I will be asking you a few questions."

The son was, as I recall, 15-years-old. He was tall and thin with dark greasy hair and a flat affect. He looked like he had not showered in a week. He sat in the chair, looking at the floor.

We shall call him Jeff as in Jeffrey Dahmer. Catch my drift?

Dad: "Ok. Let me first tell you what's going on to make it easier."

Me: "OK. Go ahead."

Dad: "I want my son to be put away for good. He is a sociopath. He has been in prison, psychiatric facilities, and half-way houses. No one will listen to me. He is going to start killing people. He has been torturing and killing animals since he was four or five years old. I am NOT taking him home ever again. A few years back, we found about 10 pairs of little girls' underwear underneath his clothes in a drawer. They all had been worn before.

93

We have no idea where or how he got those, and he won't tell us. His mother left because she couldn't take it any longer. I am remarried and last night, he tried to hurt my step-daughter while she was sleeping. I can't do this one more day. I am a police officer, and I have a full-time job. I can't be with him 24/7 to protect the world. He is crazy. He comes from a good home. My ex and I are loving, caring people. He is not. No one on either side of the family has had psychiatric issues. He has a screw loose somewhere. He was born that way. He was age four or five when he started showing signs of being crazy. I have nothing left to give him. You have to help me or someone is going to die."

Me: Not knowing what to say or do next. I was absolutely astonished that Jeffrey's father was talking like this in front of his son. I was sad, until the questioning began. Then sadness turned to fear.

I said to Jeffrey, "Is what your father said true?"

Jeffrey: Without missing a beat, "Yes."

Me: Hair standing up on my arms, "Do you want to kill people?"

Jeffrey: "Yes."

Me: Pausing for many seconds, trying to digest that last answer. "Do you want to hurt yourself?"

Jeffrey: "No."

Me: "Are you hearing voices telling you to hurt people?"

Jeffrey: "No. I just want to, sometimes."

Me: "Did you want to hurt your step-sister last night?"

Jeffrey: "Yes."

Me: I had nothing left to say. I wanted to vomit. I think that I recall shaking a bit at the point.

Jeffrey never looked up at me. He looked unaffected by what was happening. The father was showing despair and frustration. Jeffrey showed nothing.

All that I could think of was "How did this happen?" He came from a loving, middle class home, according to his father. Did a rotten gene slip into the mix? Was some ancestor of his, long ago, a Viking, per chance, who was raping and pillaging? No clue. Jeffrey was apparently NOT born with a clean slate.

I walked Jeffrey and his father back to the psych area and into a room. A security guard was notified of the situation and stood outside of Jeffery's door. I gave the psych social worker a "heads-up." She apparently knew Jeffrey well, and said that he had been to the hospital several times before.

It pushed sociopathic behavior to the forefront of my nightmares. Dahmer and Bundy were no longer fictional characters. They had become REAL. I had just witnessed them in person.

Onward:

I will not discount the hereditary component of psych issues like depression, schizophrenia, or bi-polar disorders. They are horrible afflictions to have to deal with. Although treatment is available, many people go off their meds or don't seek help to begin with. This can lead to a terrible existence, like divorce, homelessness, suicide, etc.

I remember this next patient like I saw him yesterday. His American parents brought him into the ER. He was a high school senior, about to graduate. His parents told me that he was adopted from China as a baby. They really had no idea of his family history.

They also told me that their son was a genius. He was graduating #1 in his senior class and was headed off to college on a full scholarship.

Let's call him Russell (after Russell Crowe in **A Beautiful Mind**.)

I saw on the triage sheet that he was "hearing voices."

Me: "Hi Russell. I am your nurse, Robin. Your intake paper says that you are hearing voices. Is that true?"

Russell: "Yes, it is."

Me: "What are they telling you to do."

Russell: "I try not to listen to them, but they are telling me to do weird things. I won't do it."

Me: "What kind of weird things are they saying."

Russell: "I don't know. It's not all the time, but it is getting worse. They wanted me to punch someone for no reason. I won't do that."

This was way above my scope of practice. I opted to let the family know that a psych social worker would be in to talk with them ASAP.

Russell touched my heart. He was gentle and kind. He just wanted the voices to stop. Russell did not choose schizophrenia, I assure you.

How about choices to do "street drugs?" Doing drugs to dull reality or doing drugs for pure pleasure has the same ultimate effect. Those "enjoyable drugs" can cause psychological issues, from depression, to violent tendencies, to paranoia, etc.

I have always declared that we are all one sperm and egg away from being born to a drug-addicted mother and a child-molesting father.

And so: NATURE VS NURTURE: The reasons one can blame for being nuts.

I think that both play a role in one's psychological health and wellness, or lack thereof.

More importantly, I don't believe that the medical community, local and state governments, or laws on this planet, are keeping up with the demands needed to treat people with psychological issues. I can't give you the ultimate solution other than to say, **"Something needs to be done, immediately."**

There is one place that people who need any sort of psychological help, can go: THE HOSPITAL…and they do.

More and more humans with psychiatric issues are turning up in the hospital for emergent care. Understandable. Where the heck else can they go? They have no other choice.

And so, moving on, ceasing my rant for a moment, here are just a few more of my encounters with psych patients:

One never forgets their first.

This is how I remember that day:

I was in my early 20s, in nursing school, doing my first required psych rotation.

For some unknown reason, my instructor decided to put four of us "virgins", on day one of our psychiatric clinical class, in the "locked down" psych unit of one of the largest intercity hospitals in this country. All of us looked about 14 years old, even though we were in our early 20s.

The door to get into this crazy place, was made of metal and probably weighed as much as a car. We were guided into the main psych day room by the same woman who played the nurse in **One Flew Over the Cuckoo's Nest**, or so it seemed.

The four of us moved together as one unit, floating in space and time. The door slammed shut behind us and automatically locked. We all jumped in unison. I could instantly hear my heart racing in my ears, at about 200 MPH. Was this how I was destined to die?

"Nurse Ratched" pointed over to four seats against a wall and firmly stated, "Go sit over there."

And so, we did, and I began praying to God that I would not be murdered by a lunatic, that this would all be over in less than one hour, and that I would be able to tell my mother, one more time, how much I loved her.

Here we were, four very naive "youngins," looking like four deer staring into headlights. My eyes, scanning the room, saw a catatonic woman lying on a gurney, a young girl with long blond hair, who was leaping and grasping at seemingly nothing in the air, and a man, crouched down with his hands over his head, just to name a few. I felt like we were watching a scary movie, awaiting a horrific scene to happen.

I don't believe any of us nursing students were actually breathing. I felt like this horror flick was never going to end. Was the teacher ever coming back? I prayed harder.

All of a sudden, the man who had been crouched down, stood up, dropped his arms by his side, and looked straight into my eyes. He immediately came running towards me, at full speed, across the room, yelling at the top of his lungs, "INCOMING," and crawled under my chair. I leaped up and stood on the chair, shaking to death.

Fortunately, a very large, African-American, male tech, who could have played defensive tackle for the Miami Dolphins, slowly walked over to me and helped me off the chair. I wanted to kiss him for saving my life. He then lifted the chair up and helped "George" to stand up as well, calmly stating, "Come on George, the war is over."

He put the chair back down and placed George under the table in the middle of the room, where George seemed to relax. I didn't relax at all. At least not until our teacher returned to collect us, about 30 minutes after the event. It felt like 30 hours, really.

I was certain, on that day, that I would never be a psychiatric nurse. Little did I know that EVERY NURSE IS A PSYCHIATRIC NURSE. I still have PTSD from that day.

Next topic:

Substance abuse is an epidemic in this country. That is not a secret. It not only affects the humans doing it, but also their families. Hospitals, clinics, jails, prisons, psychiatric facilities, substance abuse treatment centers, etc. are severely impacted with these people who choose drugs, including alcohol, over a clean and productive life, for whatever reason.

After reading article after article on the effects of drugs and alcohol on the brain, it is clear to me that substance abuse ultimately can cause memory loss, dementia, seizures, depression, anxiety, insomnia, etc. Taking care of this group over the years only solidifies the research. Doing drugs is an active choice, and it is a bad choice for multiple reasons, including horrible, long-lasting consequences.

Next case:

I was given a nursing assignment, one sunny day, that included taking care of an amphetamine addicted patient. He had frequented our ER, but I never had the pleasure of taking care of him. We shall call him Mr. Meth.

A very nice security guard sat outside his room. Patient Meth sat on the bed. There was nothing other than the bed was in the room, due to this patient's violent history.

I went cheerfully into the room and introduced myself. The security guard walked in the room behind me:

Me: "Hello Mr. Meth. I am Robin, your nurse. I will be taking care of you today. Is there anything you need right now?"

Mr. Meth: He stood up from the bed and raced towards me, like a bat out of hell, while yelling at the top of his lungs, **"I AM GOING TO KILL YOU RIGHT NOW."**

Me: Quickly, actually in flight, I exited the room.

Mr. Security Guard yelled for help, and he immediately stopped Mr. Meth Head from KILLING ME. OMG!

Four Security guards were able to get crazy Meth Head back into bed and calmed down without restraints. I love those peeps.

I was banned from that room and so was every other little female for that matter.

Another nurse saved by a security guard!

I surmise that Mr. Meth was born with a clean slate and opted to muck that slate up. (My story, anyway.) I am also hopeful that he eventually accepted some sort of treatment. Yep, I am an eternal optimist.

Here is a statistic for you: According to the **Journal of Clinical Nursing**, about 20% of all nurses' struggle with an addiction to drugs or alcohol.

Other research studies that I read from 2024 stated 18% of nurses show signs of substance abuse problems, while one-third of this population had a full-blown substance use disorder.

Sad.

I was a traveling nurse on a post-op unit in a Western state. It was around 1991. It was my first day on the job. I was assigned 10 post-op patients with the help of a nursing assistant. I worked 3:00-11:00 P.M.

It was a horrific first night. I worked my tail off. Most of my patients were on post- op day #1, and thus, they required a lot of attention.

It was in the days of paper charting, and so I didn't finish my shift until 1:00 A.M. I was exhausted.

My next 3:00-11:00 P.M. shift went something like this:

Another nurse at 3:00 P.M. walked up to me and stated, "Our manager wants to see you in her office right now."

Me: "FUC-!" (Thinking: Is that ever good? Anyone have a manager call you into the office for something wonderful? Pretty rare.)

Manager: "Hi Robin. Welcome to our hospital. How are things going?"

Me: Thinking to myself: WTH? What did I do? Please God, don't let her tell me that I am fired. Even worse, please don't have her tell me that I killed someone.

Me: "Everything is fine. I was busy last night. Is everything ok?"

Manager: "Well that is why I wanted to talk to you."

Me: "Ok." Thinking: Please shoot me. Let's just get this over with.

Manager: "Did you have to medicate all of your patients for pain when you arrived on your shift yesterday?"

Me: "What?" I was very confused as to what she was asking me.

Manager: "Were your post-op patients in a lot of pain when you initially assessed them?"

Me: (Thinking: Is this a trick question?) "Yes. They were post-op. They required pain medication. Is there a problem?"

Manager: "Well, Robin. A large amount of Morphine went missing yesterday."

Me: (Thinking: I want my mommy!)

Manager: "Did you get report from Nurse Janis Joplin yesterday?" (Name change)

Me: "Yes. Yes, I did. She is also a traveling nurse, right? She was very nice."

Manager: "Yes. She is a traveling nurse from another company. She has been here a few days, Robin. The pharmacy notified us that the morphine count was off yesterday after the day shift, and so we have been investigating why that happened."

"I talked extensively with all the patients you both took care of. They all said the same thing. They all concurred that Janis was acting oddly. They were in terrible pain until you arrived and medicated them. They all spoke highly of you. Thank you."

Me: Stunned. Shocked. And most importantly relieved.

I had never before worked with a nurse who had been addicted to anything other than fun. Maybe I just wasn't looking for that. How could she let those people suffer? I know now that addiction is a very selfish disease. It certainly affects one's judgement.

Anyway. Janis confessed to taking the morphine and was immediately let go from that job. Hopefully, they got her some help.

I remember several other psych patients that I took care of over the years:

There was a pedophile man who lived with his mother. He frequently tried to kill himself by cutting razor blades in quarters and swallowing them. He kept coming to our ER stating, "I want to die. I ate a razor blade." Did it ever kill him? Not that I am aware of. He ended up moving out of the area.

My career has taught me that only wonderful humans die way too young. The rotten ones hang onto this planet forever. Maybe they just have more lessons to learn.

Next:

It was early on in my career. I was trying to calm down a "Looney Tooney," 70ish-year-old female with a long history of psych issues. A male nurse was assisting me.

She was in a four-bed ward. Each bed maintained its so-called privacy with the infamous, green, curtain around it.

Ms. L. Tooney had urinated all over her bed. We had to change the linens. The plan was to stand her up, walk her to the bathroom, and help her get cleaned up while one of us changed the sheets.

Her very strange son, also a Loony Tooney, was sitting in a chair next to the bed. He was a clone of a character from **One Flew Over the Cuckoo's Nest**:

He was approximately 50 years old. He was living with his mom. Son of Ms. Loony Tooney was not working due to being "under psychiatric care," according to him. The apple definitely "did not fall far from the tree," in this case.

We had the curtain pulled around us. We were explaining to Ms. Tooney exactly what we would be doing.

Suddenly, without provocation, she began screaming at the top of her lungs: "Get that thing out of my vagina, now. Ouch! Ouch! Stop pushing that thing in me." The yelling and accusations continued.

Son Tooney "tried" to calm his mother down, which consisted of him saying in a whisper, "Mom, calm down." And then he sat down and that was his contribution.

I could hear the other patients whispering. I peeked around the curtain, and there were three women standing close by and staring at me, looking terrified.

"Everything is okay," I said. "She is just a bit confused." That was the understatement of the decade.

She was walked to the bathroom, cleaned up and the sheets were changed. Throughout this process, she continued to accuse us of unspeakable things that she must have experienced in the past. My guess anyway.

After the clean-up, we transferred her to another unit, into a private room.

I went home that night very sad. Did this woman experience sexual abuse at a younger age? Was her weird son doing awful things to her? Was her behavior a psychotic break? Did those horrible things push her into psychological distress, or was she born a Looney Tooney?

I am not a psychiatrist, so I couldn't diagnose her sudden outburst. But I definitely saw two different personalities in one human that evening.

The next day, I called the unit Ms. Tooney was transferred to, and I spoke with the nurse taking care of her. I asked how LT was doing. The nurse insisted that Ms. Tooney was oriented and doing "just fine".

She had not uttered another insane rant in the past 24 hours. They considered her a lovely and cooperative patient. The unit had no record of her son coming to see her or any visitor for that matter.

Really? Well then, maybe I had a nightmare.

Moving on, let's not leave out trauma from a horrible life of molestation, rape, abuse, etc. That would knock anyone down to the ground. It's enough to make anyone go nuts or consider suicide to escape the reoccurring visions and nightmares.

Suicide is on the rise. There were over one million suicide attempts in 2020 according to The American Foundation for Suicide Prevention. The CDC stated that suicide rates increased approximately 36% between 2020-2021. According to the World Health Organization, an estimated 703,000 people a year take their own life from around the world. How horrible is that?

And so, I decided to take a class on forensic nursing. I learned about taking care of victims of violence, conducting a thorough forensic exam, collecting evidence, etc. The instructor talked about suicide. It was a wonderful, insightful lecture.

About one week later, I was assigned to a teenager who had frequented the ER with suicidal attempts. She was not only physically beautiful, but so was her gentle spirit. I had taken care of her before. I remembered her. She remembered me. Her "method of destruction" was cutting her wrists, superficially. Let's call this patient Marilyn Monroe.

Her mother was the one who always brought her into the ER. The whole situation made Mom sad, and she expressed feelings of despair. I promised both of them that I was there to help.

I felt so empowered now, after taking that forensic class. I was given the tools to handle this situation. I would go into the room and conduct a thorough survey, as taught to me. I would get to the bottom of this.

Here is about how it went:

(Mom was in the waiting room. There was a security guard outside of Marilyn's room preventing any more suicide attempts.)

Me: Walking into the room: "Hi Marilyn. My name is Robin. I am your nurse and I will be taking care of you."

Marilyn: "Hi. I remember you. You are nice."

Me: "I remember you too, Marilyn. How are you feeling right now?"

Marilyn: "I'm okay, I guess."

Me: "Do you still want to hurt yourself?"

Marilyn: "No."

Me: "Do you want to die, Marilyn?"

Marilyn: "Sometimes."

…and the suicide/forensic questioning continued as per the class. I felt so knowledgeable and therapeutic. I felt like I could solve this puzzle.

Me: "Is someone hurting you? You can tell me, Marilyn. I want you to feel safe. I want you to have a wonderful life. I want to help you."

Marilyn: She paused for a long while, staring down at the bed. Time stopped. It felt like 10 minutes went by. Finally, looking right into my eyes, Marilyn said, "Yes. My dad has been sexually molesting me since I was five years old, and I want it to stop. Please don't tell my mother. It would kill her."

Me: Nothing. Complete silence filled the room. You could have heard a pin drop. I had no words. I felt my face turn bright red. I became deeply saddened and angry. How could anyone molest this perfect, young, "cheezit"? I was going to throw up.

Then it hit me all of a sudden. My mood changed. I became scared.

Marilyn started to cry.

What do I do now?

I had taken this wonderful class that taught me how to figure things out, BUT NOT WHAT TO DO WITH THE INFO.

A perfect example of "You don't know what you don't know, but you think you know." One of my mantras was turning back onto me. UGGG.

This perfect child had opened up to me, and I had no clue what to do next but hug her until she pulled away and thanked me for listening.

Suddenly, I remembered that I was not in this war alone.

I stood up and told Marilyn that I would need to share what she had told me with the psych social worker. She agreed and again begged me not to tell her mother. I opted to punt that request to the psych social worker, and I told the patient so.

I don't remember the end result. I do remember that the psych person was one of the nicest social workers in town. She was the perfect person to handle this situation delicately.

This story obviously stuck with me. It gets me emotional to even tell you about it. A sweet child being molested by a parent or anyone makes me sick.

I absolutely understand why living was hell for her. I just wanted to make it all better.

From that point on, I would tell anyone that I trained, "I have only a small amount of knowledge, but I will teach you what I know. Experience is the best teacher. Time spent in the nursing profession is research on a daily basis. The learning never ends."

"Every day is a school day."

And…most importantly:

9 8 8 is the phone number to call for the Suicide and Crisis Lifeline.

Please Help Me!

There are so many essential workers in a hospital. I am not sure why only nurses and doctors get that title. If only those two professions existed in the medical realm, then healthcare would shut down immediately.

The line "It Takes a Village" is exactly true when it comes to the inner workings of a medical facility. No one job can stand alone. We all rely on each other to care for the sick and to deal with humanity.

On my planet, anyone who works in a hospital, or in the medical profession, is an essential worker. Patients need us and medical people need each other.

In this chapter, I will only talk about five of these essential workers. However, there are many more.

Security guards:

This world is a crazy place with some very crazy people in it. Therefore, one of the most essential employees who deal with nutty humans in a hospital today are the security guards.

Security guards are definitely needed to keep unruly personage at bay, in any facility. Humans who are nuts and can go bonkers at any moment, can be equated to earthquakes: No one has a clue when the world will start shaking, followed by mayhem.

I have many, many experiences with the security department coming to my rescue at work. I am 5'2" and incapable of defending myself from a crazy, 6-foot male, methamphetamine user, with super strength. I know my limitations.

I have many of my own personal stories about living with the security clan. This next story happens to be my favorite. The security guard and I are still friends, years later. Let's just call him THE HULK.

This Hulk, in my mind, is nine feet tall and six feet wide. He can lift up a house. In spite of his intimidating size, he is absolutely a gentle giant. The Hulk is soft spoken, kind, and caring. He has a beautiful and sweet wife as well. I am indebted to him forever and ever. Here is why:

In the ER's where I have worked, there is always a designated section for the psych patients. A security guard stands outside of a psych patient's room in this area, in order to "keep the peace."

On this particular day, for reasons that still make me shake my head, I was assigned to an autistic, 6-foot teenager, with severe anger issues. Bear in mind that my weight, at that time, was about 120 pounds and again, I was 5'2". I was very happy that the security team "had my back" and my front and sides as well.

The patient (let's be respectful and just call him THE PATIENT) was placed in and out of restraints, depending on his behavior at any given moment.

(Side note: I have worked with autistic children since I was nine years old and I volunteered at their school several times during my years in elementary school. I still have a soft spot for them and their families, despite this story.)

The patient had been residing with us for months in the ER. Yes, MONTHS IN THE ER, as the state was trying to find him placement, a difficult task, because The Patient could go from sweet kid to insane, "rabid dog," in a second. Gut-wrenching on so many levels.

Anyway, I had gone into his room. As I was talking to him gently, while he was lying in bed, he went coo coo. He kicked me with all of his might and sent me backwards into a wall. Security guard HULK and others ran into the room and put him back into restraints. The patient was reassigned to a much larger male nurse. Thank goodness.

Speed forward to a few hours later:

The same patient had been taken out of restraints. He was calm and eating his lunch. I was charting on a computer which was located down the hall from his room.

All of a sudden, The Patient, with an insane look in his eyes, ran out of his room at full speed, towards me. I felt my life flash before my eyes, when out of nowhere (actually out of the heavens) appeared THE HULK.

The Hulk lifted up The Patient and got him to his room without incident. What I mean by that is, that The Hulk prevented The Patient from CAUSING MY DEATH.

Tears. The Hulk became my forever hero.

Now, I dare you to tell me that the security team of men and women are not essential workers. Hell, they are the MOST ESSENTIAL WORKERS.

The Housekeepers

Who the heck, in their right mind, would sign up to annihilate the bugs in a hospital that come out of every hole in a human being? Seems like combat pay would be in order.

Yes, as a nurse I am on the front lines. I have been pee peed on, pooped on, vomited on, etc. I have cleaned myself up and the patients as well. But housekeepers have to actually scrub off volumes of that yuck from all over patient rooms, in hallways, on floors, and on walls of a hospital. Ewww! How the heck do they remain so cheerful? I would be spending ½ of my day saying, "What the hell is this? And, "Grossssss!" And, "That stinks." And, "I need a shower, immediately." And, "I am taking the next job available in the cafeteria."

I have worked with the most wonderful housekeepers who have spent hours, not only cleaning up after patients, but also cleaning up after staff members who miss the garbage can, leave their trash from lunch on the counters, and virtually leave the nurses station or the doctor's office a mess.

Housekeepers are like mothers and fathers, cleaning up after lazy teenagers. Hopefully, CEOs are reading this book and are about to comply with my recommendation that all housekeepers working in the healthcare industry, get a $100-an-hour raise. They deserve it.

What? Do you want to do that job? I didn't think so.

Next: **The Kitchen Staff**. Gosh, what a great crew.

I have worked in some hospitals that have served the most incredible 5-star meals. They offered a multitude of options, from a hot meal, to a salad bar, to the usual deli-style burgers, fries, and sandwiches. Yummy.

My favorite meals were at a prominent University Hospital in Northern California. I worked a 12-hour shift and never brought food from home. My lunches and dinners were eaten with delight at that facility. No one ever sent out for food. Why would they?

So, I have a theory. (I actually have many theories, but this one is relevant to the topic that I am discussing): NEVER TELL ANYONE AT WORK, THAT YOU LOVE THE FOOD IN THE CAFETERIA, or that you love anything at work, because it will disappear.

I hardly ever brought my lunch to work in the early 2000's. Why, you ask?

Here is the story:

Once upon a time, there was this wonderful Asian family who prepared the meals for the staff and visitors, at a hospital in Northern California. It was the most delicious, pleasing, and flavorful food ever. On Fridays, the family always served a wonderful fish dish plus burgers, fries, hotdogs, and many other options. The food they created far exceeded any other generic food.

The cafeteria at lunch and dinner time, was a meeting place to vent, laugh, chat, and eat well.

I recall that supper was discounted for seniors. And so, seniors, who lived even remotely close to the hospital, would come and eat a deliciously-prepared din din. They loved it. The staff loved it. Everyone loved it. We also loved the warm and friendly family who prepared and served those meals.

I would brag about the delicious food in the cafeteria to anyone who would listen, including the administrators. Horrible mistake. I would tell them what a wonderful job this family was doing in our hospital kitchen.

Where did it get me?

All of a sudden, the delicious food ceased to exist. The family preparing the food was let go, and "healthy options" appeared. I kid you not. No more greasy, yummy fries. No more delicious food. No more wonderful, mouthwatering, sensational meals. Hamster food, all flavorless options--replaced desirable, delicious meals. To top it off, the prices went sky-high.

Seniors stopped coming. Nurses started bringing their own lunches. The cafeteria became empty. It seems that the cuisine had been enjoyed far too much to keep. Yet again, I'm on the wrong planet.

Moral of the story: Don't tell anyone at work that you absolutely love something and that it is wonderful. It will disappear and be replaced by something cheaper, less appealing, and definitely by a barely usable option. (That is from my personal research, anyway.)

Onward.

The Engineers and Mechanics:

The engineers or mechanics are the men and women who fix broken stuff in a hospital. I am very happy that they exist. Can you image if we had to call any outside repairman to come and deal with the issue at hand?

I have absolutely no idea how to fix a broken bed, a non-working IV pump, or a tube system that refuses to send a tube when you press GO.

Engineers and mechanics are worth their weight in gold.

While I do appreciate those repairmen and women, and I let them know that, these essential workers seem like robots to me. None of them ever smile or introduce themselves. They walk around with a tool belt, staring straight ahead, looking like they are on a mission to repair the space shuttle.

They are essential peeps. Things are always breaking down in a hospital. We need them.

But it is not that easy to just call engineering when something breaks down in the hospital. You have to know, by osmosis, if the broken item falls under the category of "engineering" or "biomed." You probably know where I am going with this.

If you call engineering to fix a broken piece of equipment, you most certainly will be at the wrong address and will be instructed to call biomed. That starts the wave of filling out a red or pink tag with tons of info, including your bra size, and putting that tag on the broken piece of equipment, with no promise that Mr. Biomed will ever get to it this month. I swear that I am not exaggerating. I also swear that my posse is laughing while reading this section.

Here is an example: Let's just say that a bed is stuck in the up position. The patient needs to use the bathroom. This would now require the help of an engineer to repair the bed or we'd need to purchase a parachute for the patient.

And so, this starts the process of notifying the "correct address" by calling, tagging, writing down numbers, etc. etc. It could take anywhere between ten minutes to three more phone calls to get Mr. Mechanic to the room where the broken bed lives. (A parachute seems quicker and more time-efficient to me, but we wait for the repair guy or gal.)

In reverse, because nurses have so much free time to go on this quest of assistance, (I say jokingly) if you call biomed, you will probably be told to call engineering.

It is a pot shoot. Flip a coin.

If my coffee was perfect at 6:00AM and I didn't hit any red lights on my way to work, I know that my first guess of calling engineering would be correct. When your day starts out wonderfully, everything falls in order.

Bottom line: I am happy there are essential workers of the "fixing" kind.

Supply Clerks:

These are the employees who can tell you where stuff is, where it has been moved to, how to get stuff, how to order stuff and honestly, if you will ever see that stuff again. They are also the ones who find fiendish pleasure in secretly moving supplies around according to where they THINK any random supply should be.

The supply room of every department, in a hospital, on this planet, is forever being revamped, reorganized, and redone. (God forbid you leave stuff in the same place for more than a week. The staff will actually be able to find it. What fun is that?)

Occasionally, if I needed a supply from the supply room, I would announce to the staff in the patient room at the time, that I was "heading out on a scavenger hunt and I'd hoped to win." I actually got a laugh off of that statement, a few times.

One day, a new manager showed up and reorganized our storeroom for the 6378th time. At this particular time, the reorganization of the storeroom finally seemed logical.

Every item was put into its own labeled bin, on a shelf. Each shelf represented a system, i.e., GI, OB, Cardiac. So, if I needed an NG tube, (nasogastric tube) I would head to the GI cart and find it. Perfect.

No one took into consideration that different supply clerks appear frequently in the ED. Some clerks were young enough to be my children; some were young enough to be my grandchildren; and many had no clue that this particular reorganization of our store room, took months to accomplish.

Here was one storeroom event in my life:

On this particular day, the young supply clerk walked into the store room to refill the bins. Let's call her Juno because I love that movie and my young rescue dog is named Juno as well.

I don't remember the item that I was searching for in that storeroom, but I did call it by its real name, when I talked with Juno. For the sake of reenacting this little skit, let's call that supply a "chee chee."

Me: (I had just spent five minutes trying to locate that chee chee.) "Hi Juno. Any idea where the chee chees have been moved to? They are not where they usually are."

Juno: (FYI, she did look 16-years-old.) "What's a chee chee?"

Me: (I gave her a detailed description and even pulled up a photo on my phone of an actual chee chee.)

Juno: "OOOOO! I moved it over here."

Me: (Sighing. Juno had moved a GI item to the respiratory cart.)

Juno again: "Sometimes the bins don't fit on a shelf, so I just move them where they will fit."

Me: "Well, that explains a whole lot, Juno." (Aha! Now I understand why getting a supply is always a fox hunt.)

"May I ask, did you get any formal training for this job?"

Juno: "Yes."

Me: "Ok. Let me add something to your training if I may. Each bin has to stay on the shelf that it was born on. Long ago, this room was reorganized and little bins were permanently placed in certain spots. If you move them, we nurses have no idea where to find certain supplies. Did that help?"

Juno: "Yes, it did. No one told me that. I have been moving bins since I started."

Me: "Yep. I am aware. Thanks for helping me, Juno. You have a nice day." Sigh.

Fortunately, for many years, a perfect angel was our supply clerk. She was older and experienced. We loved her. We worshipped her. The storeroom was immaculate 100% of the time that she worked. We could find everything, and if we couldn't she definitely would…in seconds. But the ER is a crazy place with an insane number of varied supplies, and that means a ton of work for a clerk. That supply angel opted to move to a slower department. I can't blame her.

P.S. I don't think Juno was the only one playing pranks on the staff without knowing it. I am hopeful that she took my advice to leave the bin where it was."

One small step for Juno, one giant leap for nurses who are looking for supplies.

You Are Essential, Too

Suppose you consult the **Webster's Dictionary**, the **Oxford Dictionary**, or me. In that case, we all concur that the word "essential" means necessary and important, like water or heat or a really good pen to write with or coffee ice cream. I have thus, labeled several more occupations in the hospital as essential to nurses. Without these peeps, I am 100% certain that nurses would be assigned to do their jobs.

Since every nurse on this planet is overworked, I am pretty sure that 100% will agree with me when I say, "Please keep your jobs; you other essential workers. We don't want to do any part of it. We are busy enough." (Well, maybe 95% of nurses are overworked and certainly at least one won't agree with ANYTHING that I say.)

Here are a few other essential people who I personally value. (There are many, many more, but I won't have a chance to mention them all. Sorry. I still appreciate your hard work and I deem you essential.)

I will now cover the "necessary employees" who affected my life in the hospital setting. They are the working crew that I couldn't live without, and thus, they shall be named: "Some of Robin's most essential workers." (In no particular order.)

The Loading Dock Guys/Gals:

I am NOT unloading an 18-wheeler full of hospital supplies. That is where I draw the line as a nurse. Nurses have already been given the responsibility of moving very obese patients by themselves, around the hospital, pushing heavy equipment here and there, and moving hospital beds from one place to another. You wonder why most nurses, at some point in time, have back issues. (My personal research.)

The hospital needs supplies to function + truck needs unloading = Essential Loading Dock Peeps. (Algebra for the umpteenth time.)

Go on with your bad selves, loading dock people. You ARE essential.

The Painters:

Not a bad gig, if you ask me. You start at one end of the hospital and paint your way to the other end.

At that point, it's time to start over again. (Kind of like the Golden Gate Bridge crew.) Nobody bothers you because nobody really notices you. Low stress and definitely a consideration in my next life.

It would not be a good idea to add this job to the job description for nurses. You see, painting would be low on the priority list. Save someone's life or paint? Give IV antibiotics or paint? Eat lunch or paint? Get what I am saying?

Essential worker (or me in my next life): The Painters.

The Techs:

Once upon a time, before most of you were born, nurses were told that there was going to be a new profession known as "techs." We "fought" against it. We were all afraid that they would take our jobs. We felt like we were losing control of our profession.

What the hell were we thinking? They were a gift from God.

Techs help us with EVERYTHING, from taking patients to X-ray or MRI; to helping us turn and clean an incontinent patient; to helping doctors during a procedure; to splinting a broken bone; etc. Their job description probably ends with "etc. etc."

We did all of those things by ourselves, long, long ago. But administrators have added 3867 jobs to the nurse's job description this year alone, I believe. There is absolutely no possible way that nurses could achieve their daily expectations without the assistance of techs.

You gave us nurses a taste of "help" in the form of another human, called techs. When one of them doesn't show up to work, due to an illness, or a car accident, or they are sick and tired of the nurses' demands on them, we are lost. We fumble around. We complain a lot. We weep.

By taking some responsibilities off of the nurses, nurses are able to do the job for which they were trained.

Techs are beyond essential to the workflow in a hospital. They are Essential XXL!

The Unit Secretaries:

God bless these essential humans. Technology changes so fast; yet, they are able to adjust like no tomorrow.

I once tried making a "recheck doctor's appointment" for a discharged patient. Sounds easy, but it is virtually impossible without a week's worth of training. I ain't got that kind of time.

Unit secretaries are able to accomplish anything needed, from taking payments, to making follow-up doctor's appointments, to ordering pizza for lunch. They amaze me. How can they be so consistently knowledgeable and efficient without missing a beat?

I did find one fault…and I mean ONLY ONE FAULT with these essential workers. They frequently forget that names repeat themselves. Many units within the frame of a hospital, have 7-Johns, 6-Julies, 5-Jims, 4-Justins 3-Jennifers 2-Jaimes (pronounced the same but spelled two different ways) and 1 Anastasia.

For example:

Frequently, the unit secretary would announce overhead, "John, pick up on line two please." Obviously, this would cause a stampede, as 7 guys, named John, would jog (or walk fast) to answer a phone call, from possibly their wife, or their lover, or the X-ray department, asking them to come get their patient now, or Home Depot, telling them that their order has arrived at the store. Imagine their frustration after picking up the phone, and finding out that they were the wrong John.

This happened to me, and other humans on the job, 487,569 times a year. At least it felt like that.

When I tired of disbanding what I was doing at the time of those pages overhead, I finally pulled rank. I stopped answering any phone calls. I let my other name-sake answer it. That worked for a while, until guilt set in. Then, after a few years, whoever was able, answered the call. Sometimes neither of us opted to answer any calls on that particular day.

Passive aggressive? YES! Passive aggressive behavior because we were sick and tired of hearing, "Robin, pick up on line five." We would then have to pick up the phone and overhead page, "Which Robin?"

FYI unit secretaries: God created last names for just that purpose.

Bottom line. It's the simplest things that often mess us up.

And still…Unit secretaries are essential to ME.

Physical Therapists, Occupational Therapists, Speech Therapists:

These are very specialized workers. Their job is to get the patient moving. Stand them up. Help them learn to walk all over again. Teach them to speak again. Help them to be able to take care of themselves.

You want someone who has lots and lots of time to teach patients. These workers are devoted to their craft and definitely essential. Nurses don't have time to devote to these things anymore.

For example, in order to be a physical therapist, you have to really want the job. A physical therapy degree requires grueling college training.

Most of them attended school longer than nurses, in order to obtain their degree. They have to have an undergraduate four-year degree in something like biology or psychology. At that point, when they have had absolutely enough of school and are teetering on the option of becoming an ice cream store owner, they have three more years to go, to get their Doctor of Physical Therapy. That is seven long years of college.

In the hospital, we depend on these physical therapists. I gained personal respect for them, just watching them slowly work with sick patients, as they'd get them gently out of bed and upright. I have watched physical therapists work with post-surgical patients, hip fractured people, weak humans, unsteady humans, etc. That job takes patience, kindness, strength, and tenacity. Maybe it is just luck, but I have not met a rude therapist yet.

Here is a story for you. This particular story has repeated itself about 8,924 times in my career:

One day, when I was just a puppy in the field of nursing, a patient of mine needed assistance to go to the bathroom. She refused a bedside commode. She refused a bedpan. She felt too embarrassed to use any items to pee or poop into, in the same room with another patient. She refused to use the walker because, "I am too weak and I have to have a BM NOW!"

It was in the early days of my career, when everyone told me what to do, and I did it. (That changed pretty quickly.)

Let's call this patient Mama. She reminded me of Eunice Higgins's mother on **The Carol Burnett Show**. She even yelled at me the way Mama yelled at Eunice.

Mama took care of herself at home and used a walker to get around. She lived with her husband who she bossed around the same way she was bossing me. She told me so.

Mama kept pushing me away as I attempted to get her in the sitting position. It took a long time to simply gain her confidence and assure her that I would not let her fall. Mama had a vice grip on my upper arms as I swung her around to sit on the edge of the bed.

The algebra from this tale: Mama was big + I am little = My back issues started way back then.

Of course, there was no human to help me, so I slowly stood Mama up and pivoted her into the wheelchair. I asked her how she did this alone at home. Her response: "I do just fine, thank you."

Physical therapy was to see her that afternoon, of course. But she couldn't wait. She needed to "go to the bathroom immediately."

I wheeled her into the bathroom and stood outside the door, per her insistence, for another 10 minutes, waiting for her to finish. She promised not to stand up without calling me first. I was afraid she would fall, so I kept asking her if she was okay.

I finally got Mama back to bed. That whole scenario took almost an hour to complete. The minute the sheet was pulled up over her body, she stated, "Get me up again. I need to pee this time." UGGG!

She needed physical therapy for sooo many reasons. She came into the hospital with a urinary tract infection and weakness. She used a walker at home but the second she got to the hospital, she couldn't sit up without assistance, let alone use the walker. She was supposed to be discharged that day, of course.

The physical therapy crew ARE ESSENTIAL TO NURSES:

I had three other patients who I had not seen, as of yet. I needed to make sure that they were ok. I also needed to work more with Mama to see if she could actually use her walker. (Classic case of a nurse always having 87 things to do at once.)

How was I going to send her home if she couldn't use that walker? I needed a physical therapist to evaluate Mama and help her with her mobility issues. I had no more time to do that.

I needed that essential physical therapist.

I called the PT department to see if they could come immediately. Fortunately, someone did come. The physical therapy "angel" insisted that Mama use her walker and then guided her back to the bathroom. Mama even waved at me as she passed by.

The physical therapist had the time, energy, and strength to deal with Mama. That's her job. I wished that I had more time, but I didn't, and I still don't.

…and so, I am elated that physical therapists exist, for they are certainly an essential part of my world.

Xray Techs:

What a great job. Two years of an accredited school for radiology, and voila, you have a wonderful career.

Let's just say you love photography as well. You hit the jackpot, son.

These peeps take pictures all day long. What's the stress? "Oops. Your knee film needs to be repeated. It was a little bit far to the left."

BAM! One second later, a new picture of your left knee is done.

"Next patient."

Taking photos of the inside of humans is probably like being on a treasure hunt. I am certain that they have many stories about "funny finds."

They are essential workers. Do you know why? Because nurses have enough on their plate and don't want to add "X-ray tech" or "can take X-ray's" to their job description.

Discharge Planners:

The discharge planner is a nurse or social worker who figures out what a patient will need when they leave the hospital. The patient may be ok to go home or they may need a care facility.

The discharge planner can arrange home care services like oxygen, a hospital bed, home physical therapy, etc. They can help the patient and/or family find a care facility, for a short or long stay.

That is their job in a nutshell. They do a lot more, but we will leave it at that.

Discharge planners have huge responsibilities for typically, a zillion patients each. I have watched them over the years. They work their booties off.

When patients are told that they get to go home, these patients notoriously want all the "paperwork," plans, and implementation done NOW. I can't blame them. (By the way, the nurses, doctors and supervisors want those patients gone as well, so that their beds can be given to the next patient in line.) And so, the discharge planner is getting pressured by everyone involved.

The patient has been discharged + Discharge Planner notified = Patient goes Bye Bye ASAP. No pressure there.

Staff nurses have no time to sit on the phone waiting for medical supply people to answer and comply with items requested. Staff nurses have no time to talk with skilled nursing facilities to arrange a stay. And finally, staff nurses have absolutely NO TIME to fill out the volumes of applications and paperwork needed to get the patients the heck out of the hospital! We don't want that job added to our resume.

In short, discharge planners play a vital role in the workings of every hospital. Without them, the "go home wheel" would be much, much slower. Discharge Planners are essential workers. That's for sure.

Funny story:

A patient that I was caring for, was dying in the ER, due to end-stage alcoholic cirrhosis. In medical terms, he was "bleeding out." He was a DNR (Do Not Resuscitate).

We shall call him Mr. Jack Daniels. Jack was jaundiced. He weighed approximately 300 pounds of mostly fluid that sat in his belly from liver failure. He was taking his last breaths.

The doctor wrote an order that read: "Discharge planner to see patient ASAP to arrange a care facility."

The discharge planner sent a message back to the doctor that read:

"GOD NOTIFIED."

Get Out of Here-Now

People who are sick, are housed in a hospital. They go there for care just like a car goes to a mechanic. When the car is fixed, the car goes back home.

Why then, when human bodies are fixed, won't they go home? Once "body repairs" are completed, illness is cured, and a plan is set, isn't it time to fly away?

Apparently not.

It is as hard to get humans out of a hospital as it is to get service from any number of phone companies. (My opinion and experience as well.) You know that it will eventually happen; it just takes forever.

Let's just say that the patient has been discharged. I have completed all of the paperwork. I have picked up the discharge meds for the patient. I have dressed them, and had them brush their teeth and comb their hair. There is only one thing left to do: GET THEM OUT OF HERE-NOW.

Here are some of the actual reasons that it took so long to get my patients out of the hospital:

1. Per husband: "She can't come home. Her recliner is broken, and I don't have time to get it fixed until next week."

My thoughts: Do you not have another piece of furniture for her to sit on? Is the recliner the only furniture that is in your house? Can anyone you know help you with this issue? Do you really think we can keep patients in the hospital because of a broken recliner? Apparently, you do. Apparently, we need to build 465,365 more hospitals to keep humans inside the building until they deem they are ready to go home.

2. Per another husband: "I can't bring her home because our air conditioner is broken, and it won't be fixed for two weeks. That is when I get paid."

My thoughts: How long has this air conditioner been broken. Do you have fans? Are you having an affair and just don't want your wife home for a while?

I will tell those ten patients in the ambulance bay, waiting for a bed in the ER, that they will have to wait there for two weeks, or until the admitting physician agrees to write admitting orders for a diagnosis of "broken air conditioner."

3. Per a son: "I can't pick my mother up today. I have too many meetings."

My thoughts: Work is more important than your mother? Sad. We are not a boarding kennel. Come and get her now.

4. "You need to find me a way home!" this 22-year-old said while texting on his phone.

My thoughts: Why yes, you entitled brat. With my other 4538 jobs to do today, I will spend time on the phone finding you a way home. Have you not heard of Uber or Lyft? What is happening in this world?

5. "I don't have any money for a ride home."

My thoughts: You are a tattooed, pierced, human on your cell phone, with "no money" and you're not working, due to anxiety. Of course, the hospital will pay for you to get the heck out of here. Here you go. Here is a taxi voucher.

6. "I am not ready to go home. I want to have lunch first."

My thoughts: This situation actually happened to me several times. You'd rather have hospital food than any other food? How sad is that? We are not a restaurant. I will package your food TO GO.

In all fairness, most people do want to leave a hospital, even before they should. It is a select few who love us and our accommodations so much, that they call it their home.

In South Florida in the 1980s, on any given holiday, families would drop their elderly relatives off in the ER, with a plethora of trumped-up complaints. The family would then head out on a wonderful, planned, family vacation, and they would leave Grandma at the hospital until they returned home a week later. Of course, they didn't answer their phones, and so their stalling tactic worked. Grandma stayed with us, in the hospital, for a week.

We had more available hospital beds then. Not now.

A hospital and a hotel are similar in this way: We both only have a certain amount of space available. Once that space is used, there is no room for anyone else at "the inn".

However, the difference between a hospital and a hotel is that the population in a hospital is sick, and an available bed could mean life or death, while a healthy guest in a hotel could opt to stay forever. In fact, the hotel would certainly love an indefinite stay, but hospital staff want you out ASAP.

Let's be crystal clear: In a hospital, we want you out the minute you arrive. That is our goal: Get you well and out of our facility because there is NEVER enough room at the Hospital Inn.

So, I beg of you: When it's time to leave, LEAVE! Sick humans are waiting for your bed.

Ok, here lies the next issue:

Getting people out of the ER and into an admit bed: The patient has a bed inside the hospital, as assigned by a supervisor or bed control. Why can't we get them there? Why must we beg, plead, and threaten to tell the receiving nurse's boss or the hospital supervisor if that nurse refuses to take report? Why do we have to call, umpteen times, to get our patient out of the ER?

The hospital units must not be aware of the following: (algebra,)

There is a big hospital sign outside the building + You are a nurse = You will be getting a patient, at any moment if you have an empty bed in the area you are covering. Otherwise, the flow of patients backs up like severe constipation.

Some of the hospital nurses stall, especially the closer it gets to the end of their shift (See more reasons for stalling, below.) They would rather let the next nurse take on more patients. They have just finished discharging their patients, and they're ready to go home, ASAP. I understand. I worked inside the hospital, on various units. It gets exceptionally busy towards the end of a shift. In those days, we had no option. If the ER said you have a patient, we took that patient immediately because it was the ER. Not anymore.

A family member had been in the hospital for a few weeks. He had been discharged after having surgery.

One and a half hours after the discharge order was written, a nurse walked into the room and stated, "I am too busy to discharge you." This is the most popular stall tactic by hospital staff members (in my opinion.) That nurse then sat at the nurse's station charting for another 30 minutes until I had had enough. I called upon a familiar other nurse to "help us out" and get my relative out of the hospital. Should I have had to do that?

What those floor nurses fail to understand is we can't lock our doors in the ER. Trust me. I have suggested it many times. Humans keep flocking to the ER because they want or need medical care. As any day progresses, the ER becomes a mob environment. Help us out here people. Take your peeps.

Here are just a few of the stall tactics that I have gotten from the hospital staff when I tried to get my patient out of the ER:

1. "There is no bed in the room."

Thoughts: WTH? May I suggest that you find a bed and put it in the room that is empty and awaiting the arrival of the next patient? You know you are getting a patient. Why is there no bed in that room? Call housekeeping; or wheel an empty bed in there yourself; or call a supervisor to accomplish this task.

Note to self and to you readers: I could push a king size mattress downstairs by myself, and drag it into my trailer, and take it to the dump, 20 miles away, in the time it usually takes for a bed on wheels to be moved into an empty hospital room. Sigh.

2. "There is no nurse to take report."

Thoughts: Did I call the right place? Again, isn't this a hospital? I am happy to give report to your housekeeper for gosh sakes. (Kidding. They are busier than nurses.) Sometimes I don't get report when a patient is dropped off in the ER. Please find a nurse to take report from me.

3. "The nurse is at lunch or on break or eating somewhere or ran away as fast as possible."

Thoughts: Ran away? I sympathize. I have thought about doing the same thing on more than one occasion. Is she the only nurse on that whole unit?

Is she the only one allowed to hear what I have to say? If I just brought the patient to the room, would she refuse to care for him because I didn't give her the 411?

4. "The room is not clean."

Thoughts: This statement can result in anywhere from a five minute to three hours wait time. Trust me. I have experienced it, possibly because the housekeeper is pulled to clean 20 rooms at once. Those three housekeepers for the entire hospital (my quantity guess) work their buns off. I have volunteered more than once to go up and clean the dirty hospital room. (Against protocol apparently.)

5. "I need 10 minutes more to finish what I am doing. Can I call you back?"

Thoughts: This would be fine if it didn't happen all of the time. BTW, it is never 10 minutes. It's more like 30-60 minutes. Take the patient already.

Case in point: True story: It happened to ME.

Me: "Hello. This is Robin in the ER. I would like to call report to the nurse who will be taking care of Ms. E." (E for Exhausted waiting for a darn bed.)

Nurse T. (for Turtle.): "Hi. This is T. I am right in the middle of taking care of a patient. Can I call you back in 20 minutes?" (My thoughts: Isn't she always in the middle of taking care of a patient? I know that I am.)

Me: The scene: It was 2:30 P.M. and the ER looked like the front of Walmart on Dec. 26th at 5:00 A.M. One million people were there (or so it felt that way) and 10 ambulances were lined up out the back door, as the medics were waiting to not only give report to a nurse, but begging to off load their human. I was approaching my limit in the patience department.

I took a deep breath: "Well T., if that is the case, I will tell the 20 ambulances waiting patiently outside, that Nurse T. needs 20 more minutes. Will that work for you?"

Nurse T: "Wow. OK. I will take report."

Me: "Thanks."

Why the Heck Would You Want to Do That?

My father always wanted me to be a doctor. He told me this about 64 times a year. At least. Don't get me wrong. He was proud of me as a nurse. He just felt that I had the smarts, personality, tenacity, and stomach to handle it. I believe that he thought doctors stacked up just below God.

My dad was part of the WWII generation. He enlisted in the Air Force and flew fighters in three wars. He had the personality to be a physician but would have never been able to handle the "ewww" stuff.

Dad, like everyone from his generation, listened to, respected, and admired their doctors. They rarely questioned their diagnosis, treatments, medications, or plan of care. They had all the faith in the world that each doctor knew what he was doing.

The WWII generation showed respect, honesty, and integrity in all areas of their lives. It is what they stood for. It is why I tried, on many occasions, to confine my practice to ONLY WWII Vets. Unfortunately, that didn't happen.

And no, I never wanted to be a doctor. I am an old soul. I knew, at a young age, that it wasn't in my future. Here are some of the reasons why:

1. Four years of college is one thing. Even six is doable. But four years of undergraduate studies + four years of medical school + three to seven years to complete a residency = 11 to 15 YEARS OF COLLEGE? --UCK ME! NO WAY! I had a life to live. I had other things that I wanted to do.

2. I definitely did not have the money. I had worked two jobs just to complete four years of college. It took me 10 years to pay those loans back. If I went to medical school, I would be in debt for the rest of my time on earth. No thanks.

(BTW, I am NOT from the "me generation" and NEVER expected ANYONE to pay my loans back, except for ME. How did so many humans get so entitled? End of this rant....)

3. The buck stops with the doctors. They are 100% responsible for the medical care that they deliver.

They do all sorts of procedures on a human body that could go sideways at any time. Malpractice is forever hovering over their heads. Who would want that pressure?

4. I always wanted a house full of kids. That didn't happen, but med school would have definitely made it impossible. Most doctors don't have an 8:00 A.M.-5:00 P. M. kind of job. Long hours come with the territory. Doctors are "married" to their work. Family time is considered "liquid gold."

5. Being a doctor is a stressful and demanding job. So, I decided to be a nurse instead. How ironic is that? I remember many years ago, nursing was voted the most stressful job on this planet. (I don't remember when or where I read that.)

6. The paperwork/computer work "from hell," is enough to discourage anyone from being a doctor. It did deter me. Nowadays, doctors spend more time staring at a computer than looking into a patient's eyes.

Medicine, like any profession, "is nothing like we experienced in school." I have heard that over and over again from physicians, who, upon completing their education, have been forced to spend minimal time with their patients, complete tons of computer charting, and live at work instead of at home. "It's not what we signed up for."

7. Regulations, rules, and protocols are constantly changing. You get in your groove, and then you are told to alter it because of new laws. Lawsuits are on the rise. This makes practicing medicine scary and frustrating.

8. Humans are rotten. They try your patience. They are hard to please. They often think they know more than any medical doctor because they've read their "needed treatment" on Google. Doctors these days have to talk some patients into adhering to the correct plan of care, and that is exhausting. (Yet another reason to become a painter: little human interactions.)

And finally,

9. I prefer animals over humans. I think I was born with that trait. In fact, if you'd asked me when I was young, what I wanted to be when I grew up, I would have said, "A veterinarian." Until, of course, I realized that animals don't live as long as they should. They die young, compared to humans. How tragic. As a veterinarian, I would be crying all day long.

This, in my opinion, is one of God's few mistakes. Some humans live wayyyy too long, especially the ones with no conscience. God's animal creatures don't live long enough. By the way, in my opinion, Noah got it right: Take the animals and ditch the people.

In conclusion, in order to be a doctor, you must really, really, really love stress and torture. You must enjoy the human race at its worst. Your caring heart must be the size of Texas. It is all that I can figure out.

Alright. Let's give equal time to the "wonderful reasons to become a physician." I am struggling here, as my bias and experiences are showing. But doctors deserve this side of praise as to why they want to spend their lives doing that selfless job.

1. The ultimate altruistic job: Taking care of ill humans. With the 120,000 + jobs on this planet, (another guess), how unselfish can a person get? Doctors chose to care for the sick and injured as their career, unless, of course, they were pressured by parents and grandparents, who are all doctors. Either way, the good doctors get a gold key to enter into heaven. I am betting on that.

2. Do you love to learn new things? Want a fascinating job? This job was designed for YOU. It is a continuous brain stimulator. New medical information is constantly popping up out of nowhere. Your world at work can change in a second.

Example:

One-minute doctors are told to give a specific drug as part of the coding algorithm, and the next second, they are instructed that after years of research, "that drug" never did what it was supposed to do.

WE ARE ALL JUST PART OF ONE BIG RESEARCH EXPERIMENT! No better place to validate that statement than in medicine.

3. I still believe that physicians are labeled as one of the most trusted and honored professionals. Humans trust them with info they are too embarrassed to tell anyone else. They are the ultimate, highly-respected, leaders in healthcare. The population tends to hold these peeps in high regard, knowing how smart they must be to get where they are today.

4. Do you love lots of excitement? If so, become a doctor. As the saying goes, "One never knows what the cat will drag in." Never a dull moment.

5. There are so many opportunities in medicine as a physician, from working in a hospital, to running a clinic, to working on a cruise ship. Doctors can do research, work for a news channel or newspaper, or go into administration or public health. The list of jobs for a doctor is endless. If you get bored at your job, there are lots-o-lateral-maneuvers one can do. Not many professions can say that.

6. Doctors will have a job for a lifetime. Doctors will always be needed by the population, on this planet anyway.

Humans get sick + Humans need doctors = Job security.

7. Although I firmly believe that all those in the healthcare industry are grossly underpaid for what they do, doctors still make a good salary. They have benefits that can extend into retirement. I am pretty sure that most of them don't live paycheck to paycheck. Doctors can support their families and not go hungry.

8. Doctors Save Lives. What I mean by that is: "It Takes a Village," and physicians lead the village. One of the most amazing and rewarding benefits of being a doctor is that they can honestly state that they can save a life in an emergency. What a truly rewarding feeling. What a fantastic job.

9. Doctors teach humans how to improve their health. They are an encyclopedia of medical information. Physicians dispense that info to patients, according to their needs at the time. They are health teachers of the medical kind.

Should you go to medical school? Does the good outweigh the bad? You will have to decide that for yourselves. I made my decision and have never regretted it.

Did You Really Mean to Write That?

When you arrive at any medical care facility, doctors (or physician assistants or nurse practitioners, etc.) create orders to be carried out by the nurses, on your behalf.

The orders are like gasoline to your auto, or shall I say electricity to your hybrid electric vehicle, these days. In any case, those orders get the "show on the road." They are needed to ultimately diagnose your problem and plan your care so that you can get busy living again.

Once upon a time, there were doctors who wrote the orders with a pen. In my world, may of them did not write clearly. Any orders that nurses could not read or decipher, became game pieces. Each human on that unit, including housekeepers, was asked what they thought the writing from the doctor, said. Like any jury decision, the answer with the most votes, won. The winner was congratulated with kudos, by all involved.

Why didn't we just call the doctor to clarify his order, you ask? 99% of the time we did. It just depended on who the doctor was. Most doctors, like most people in general, are nice. But there are a few "rotten apples" in every society and profession.

In the early days of my career, a couple of the doctors, apparently took classes in how to write messy. Those same professionals learned how to be nasty and rude when asked to clarify their written orders. It was a non-punishable behavior then, for those physicians.

If you needed to call an unpleasant doctor to clarify an order, you stalled, in hopes that they would come to the unit. When that doctor arrived at the unit, you would beg any available "seasoned nurse" to speak with that doctor and clarify the order, because you were too fearful to speak with Satan.

If, by some chance, you had to call a physician at home, at night, your anxiety level would be off the charts. You would try to come up with excuses to wait until morning for clarification of that one non-urgent order.

When you finally found the guts to put in that phone call to that ill-mannered doctor with poor penmanship, he was, notoriously, condescending.

He acted like you needed to buy some reading glasses, go back to school and learn to read, or have "a real nurse" help you decode his writing. Your night would, consequently, be ruined.

In conclusion, deciphering the doctor's orders led to the patients receiving great care. However, all the nurses who practiced in the 1970s and 1980s still suffer with PTSD.

To illustrate this issue, here is a story that caused me PTSD for years, until the situation was finally handled.

In about year two of my career, as a registered nurse, I accepted the position of an assistant head nurse. There was a GI physician who worked in our facility. He was a maniac, in my opinion, and pretty much everyone's opinion who worked at that hospital. Shall we call him Dr. Evil? Yes. Let's do that.

Dr. Evil was the physician who you ALWAYS hated to call on the phone, talk to in person, or ask him any questions, ever. He was about 5'7" inches tall with dark hair. I clocked him at about 40-years-old.

Evil had a very bad temper. He yelled and threw things like his brief case or the trash can, or pens, or whatever was close to him at the time of his tantrum. (Today, he would probably be arrested or at least fired. Not then. It was in the days of doctors=Godlike. They could do no wrong, ever.)

Anyway, Doctor Evil had one too many fits on our unit, causing the sweetest nurse to cry. We all had had enough of his outbursts. Something had to be done. I had already notified our wonderful "head nurse" and the house nursing supervisor every time an event happened with Evil. They had talked with him, but to no avail.

During one dinner hour, the staff and I had a conversation about the best way to handle Dr. Evil. I believe I was the one who came up with a suggestion to curb this monster's attitude. The idea occurred to me after either reading about it or hearing from someone as a way to tame a beast of a human. The staff loved the idea and so we were all in.

The staff agreed that the next time Dr. Evil started yelling at someone, a specific word would be announced overhead along with the location on the unit of the outburst. The staff would all run to that location and encircle the rat of a doctor and start clapping in applause as loudly as we could.

And so, it was an absolutely lovely evening. Everything was going along smoothly when a very young nurse stopped Dr. Evil in the hallway. She asked him to clarify one of his written orders that she could not read. All of a sudden, Evil went bonkers and started screaming and berating this lovely RN.

I overheard the escalating conversation. I paged overhead the agreed signal. Eight nurses or so came running to the identified location. We all encircled Dr. Evil and started clapping our hands as loudly as we could. He froze in disbelief. He was stunned. Dr. Evil kept turning around inside the circle, trying to figure out what to do.

Finally, he pushed his way out of the circle and ran off the unit. I never heard him yell, scream, or be mean again.

I told our head nurse what we had done. She thought it was brilliant.

We took our power back that day. It felt good.

And so, nurses were thrilled when computer charting and ordering began. We could clearly read all the doctors' orders and notes. Hallelujah. Right?

Wrong.

Let me clarify: With the advent of computer ordering, we could clearly read each word of the order set. But sometimes, the orders made no sense at all. Computers did not stop crazy orders.

Any order could be confusing, odd, or dangerous. Deciphering the true meaning of some weird orders could be like trying to figure out what a 16-month-old baby was saying.

Again, if an order insights bewilderment, the decision-making process begins: Do I call the doctor? Do I go with what I believe the physician means? Do I wait for the doctor to arrive on the unit for clarification?

Fortunately, behaviors of physicians, in general, have changed. It is no longer deemed acceptable to throw a tantrum, yell, scream, or insult a nurse. There are avenues for reporting such conduct. Consequences for rude actions exist. Of course, may I add, "There is always one jackass."

Because of the changes in acceptable behaviors, it is very easy now to clarify orders.

Moving right along, here are some of my favorite orders over the years, written by physicians:

1. "Alert. Medication reconciliation remains incomplete, thus imperiling our opportunity to be judged to be a superior institution by external evaluators. Please rectify promptly."

This doctor thought it was the nurse's responsibility to go over the medication list of each patient when they arrived. By the way, it was the doctor's job to complete this task, that week. This job continued to be punted back and forth like a tennis ball at Wimbledon.

2. "Bipap to face." (Bipap is a non-invasive way to ventilate and support breathing, administered through a face mask.)

Very happy that the doctor ordered us to put a mask on this patient's face. I was about to place it on his knee.

3. "DC Ampicillin. DC Gentamycin and Ampicillin tomorrow and then walk to 6EB." (DC means discontinue)

This order was written by a medical student. I couldn't wait to call him for clarification. It went something like this:

Me: Hello Dr. Youngin. (We shall call this student Youngin.) This is Robin, the nurse. I need to clarify an order or two on Mrs. S. Do you want the Ampicillin DCD today or tomorrow?

Dr. Youngin: Uh, tomorrow please.

Me: Ok. One more thing. Tomorrow, after I walk to 6EB, what do you want me to do?

Dr. Youngin: Speechless.

In conclusion, I had to give him a lesson in sentence structure.

4. I am not making this next one up. I swear.

A patient arrived to the hospital in DKA. (DKA or diabetic ketoacidosis occurs when there isn't enough insulin in the body. Insulin controls blood sugar levels.) The patient's blood sugar was 294 after several insulin doses. (Per WebMD, a healthy blood glucose level on a non-fasting blood glucose test is under 125.) I sent a message to the doctor, asking him if he wanted any more insulin administered to the patient due to his continued high blood sugar level. This was his order:

"Give whatever insulin is in your syringe."

WTF? Thank God I was an experienced nurse with common sense. **Another patient saved by a nurse!** For non-medical people, insulin lowers the blood sugar. There is a significant difference between giving one unit of insulin and ten units of insulin in a syringe. Too much insulin and your blood sugar could drop fatally low.

5. "Advance diet to Regular but don't feed her if she is choking."

Drats. I was planning on holding her down and shoving food in her mouth while she was coughing up a lung.

6. "Please get the patient a pencil or pen."

In those days, we had volumes of pens at the desk. We needed them to chart. BTW, I went to nursing school to learn how to walk out of a patient's room, collect a pen, and hand it to the patient. A very useful skill, may I add. Apparently, a skill that this so-called physician did not have.

7. "Pt is still schizophrenic."

That was written as an order. Still not sure what to do with it. Didn't know that schizophrenia is like the common cold. It comes and goes!?

8. "Do not let Humpty Dumpty in the patient's room." (Made up name)

How the hell am I supposed to know who Humpty Dumpty is. I did not list police officer or FBI agent on my name tag. Was I supposed to stand guard at the door? How was I going to stop Mr. Dumpty if he was barging in? Would he fall? Would I have to complete an incident report?

I had to explain to that doctor that "bodyguard" was definitely out of my 5' 2" capabilities.

9. "Regular Diet orally."

Thank you, doctor, for writing orally on this awake and healthy woman. I was about to shove it in you know where. You absolutely saved me from embarrassment.

10. "Please make sure that her TV is set on cartoons at all times."

Sure. I have time to be on TV patrol. It was probably added to my job description that year. God knows, 487 other things had been added.

11. "Ambulate patient out of bed."

Gosh. Thanks for that order. I was planning on standing him on top of the bed and asking him to walk from the headboard to the footrest.

12. "Dysphagia diet while awake." (A dysphagia diet is used for patients who have trouble swallowing. Foods on this diet are easier to chew and swallow.)

Did that doctor think I was going to try and feed the patient while she was asleep? I'm sure glad he wrote "while awake." I would have been debating when to feed her.

13. A physician received the lab results on Steven Gestation (made-up name). At the top of the lab result page, it read, "Urine pregnancy test in lab." Apparently, someone had ordered a urine pregnancy on this male patient by mistake.
The doctor wrote a follow-up order that read, "If this patient is pregnant, I quit."

I got nothing.

14. "Change diaper if she needs it changed."

I have so much to say that I don't know where to start.

a. Nope. I was planning on changing her diaper every hour whether she needed it or not.

b. Very happy that you wrote that order. I would have just let her sit in poo until she was discharged back to the SNF (skilled nursing facility) in a few days.

c. Did you need a direct order from your wife to change your baby's diaper? Ah ha! That is why you wrote that as an order.

The list goes on....

15. "Change the patient's sheets daily."

Have you run out of order ideas? We did that anyway in those days. Do you have a clue what nurses do?

And last but not least, this doctor wrote:

16. "Please rectify. Wrong patient with these ultrasound results."

A 19-year-old male patient came to the ER with complaints of testicular pain. The ultrasound results read, pregnant uterus, perinatal, multiple gestation.

Uh oooooh!

Doctors Say the Darndest Things

Medical personnel have a very tweaked sense of humor. We acquire this peculiar trait immediately upon starting our career in the medical field. It is a necessary part of our job. Without humor, we would be in a constant state of depression. We would all need psychiatric care for life.

This strange sense of humor is a survival method. It is a shield. It is a bullet-proof curtain to hide behind. Humor diverts our mind from tragedy to anything else. Silliness keeps us upright. It allows us to get through the day without hysterically crying or screaming or yelling obscenities. Nonetheless, all three of those responses still happen periodically. Our only acceptable coping mechanism on the job is laughter.

The suffering and death, enmeshed in our jobs, take their toll on us. Sorrow chips away at every doctor, nurse, and other medical professional's soul. For the rest of society, it is like viewing **Love Story** or **The Notebook** or **Titanic** over and over again, day after day. The average person would need to purchase a pallet of Kleenex after viewing such sadness. Healthcare people use humor in place of tissues. We do sometimes use just tissues and at other times, we use both Kleenex and laughter.

Doctors and nurses have a similar weird sense of humor. We smirk and giggle at the same things. Events that would abhor the average human, bring us to tears with laughter.

I could write an entire book on the multitude of funny things that doctors have said to me during a situation that we've experienced together.

In any event, here are just a few stories that have prompted me to laugh and write them down for this book:

In the 1980s, I had a favorite surgeon who I worked with on a pre-post op unit. His name was Dr. Teddy Bear. That is what the nurses called him behind his back, anyway. It was simply because he looked like a bear and was built like a bear. But unlike bears, he had the kindest disposition of any surgeon on this planet. Unlike most surgeons at that time, he was funny and he was always in a good mood.

I was the assistant head nurse on the 3:00 P.M.-11:00 P.M. shift. Physicians sought me out to answer questions or to discuss their patients' needs. This is because the primary nurses were usually very busy. Plus, on this extra-large, 57-bed unit, it was always hard to locate a specific nurse.

On this particular day, a middle-aged woman arrived on the unit. Upon arrival, she began vomiting large amounts of red blood. (We shall call her Mrs. RBC) GI and surgery were notified of the situation and requests were made for immediate consultations.

Several nurses were frantically caring for Mrs. RBC, hoping to keep her alive until she was escorted off the unit and into surgery. They were starting IV lines, hanging blood, drawing blood, etc.

Dr. Bear arrived onto the unit, and I pointed him in the direction of the bleeding patient's room. He spent a short time in the room, realizing the need for emergent surgery to stop the bleeding.

I met Dr. Bear in the hallway outside of Mrs. RBC's room. I asked what he thought about this patient.

He thought for a moment, looked up at the ceiling and back down to me, and finally stated, "Blood outside the body is NEVER GOOD." Then he stated, "Please get her down to surgery immediately."

I and the other nurses around just laughed. What a brilliant deduction. How ingenious.

I have borrowed that quote and used it many times in my career.

Best of all, the patient went to surgery, recovered well, and went home. (Sorry, I don't recall her final diagnosis.)

Many years ago, I worked with an ER physician with his own psychological issues. We will leave it at that.

An intoxicated patient arrived in the ER. In the days of charting on paper with a pen, Dr. Odd wrote the following information under Chief Complaint:

Multiple complaints:

#1 Right hand pain after fist fighting with three guys in two days.

#2 Chronic liver pain which he is treating with daily alcohol use while operating heavy machinery.

#3 Wants more pain medication because he "had all of his clothes, tools, vitamins, and Vicodin stolen by a woman in a small car."

#4 Has "a lot of blood in his urine and poop."

By the way, this patient had driven to the ER with a blood alcohol of .21. In most states in the United States, a blood alcohol concentration level of 0.08% is considered legally intoxicated. Scary.

I have another story involving the same Dr. Odd.

A triage nurse walked over to the Dr.'s office to ask for an opinion on a patient in her triage chair. Looking for a quick response, she unfortunately selected the wrong physician. Here is how it went:

Nurse: "Could you please come out to triage and let me know if you think this laceration needs suturing?"

Dr. Odd: "Everyone has their own opinion about suturing. Some doctors prefer Dermabond. Some days, I like Dermabond too. Some doctors like to suture every laceration. Some days I do, too."

The nurse turned around in disgust and started to walk away while he was talking.

Dr. Odd: "Where are you going?"

Nurse: "I am headed back to cell block one."

An ER physician needed help with a procedure. His overhead page was "Could all available men come to room 48 now, please."

Several of us single female nurses heard the page, laughed, and walked over to that room. The doctor looked at us ladies standing outside the room and staring. I finally spoke up and stated, "For years, we have all been relying on meeting men by chance.

We were unaware that all we had to do was call for "all the available men" to a specific room.

Everyone chuckled. I wish it were that easy.

Saying "Thank You" is Just Not Enough

It just doesn't feel like enough.

-If you worked alongside some of the most brilliant minds on this planet.

-If you watched a doctor lead a team and by his commands, bring a clinically dead person back to life.

-If you witnessed a physician explain to a family, with all of the compassion and kindness he could muster up at that moment in time, that their young relative had passed away, despite the extensive efforts to save that teenager.

-If you ever saw a doctor perform a life-saving skill or procedure under the greatest pressure of time, thereby reviving that human being.

-Or if you had a physician take care of you or your family, who gave 150% by explaining the plan of care, implementing life-saving therapies, and insisting on only quality care.

…you understand that saying, "Thank you, doctor," is just not enough.

Doctors don't wear capes, like Superman or Spiderman. Some of them don't even wear white coats with their names embroidered above the left breast pocket, any longer. Short of an introduction upon meeting one of these rare creatures, they are unidentifiable in the community. They don't look any different than most humans who walk around this planet.

But they ARE different. They are super-human. Their super power is SAVING LIVES! Digest that idea for a second. Doctors can, in real life, prevent you from dying. They can bring you back to life. They can even ease you into death, without suffering or pain. If that is not a super power, what is? No wonder they are compared to GOD.

The stress that these Superheroes live with on a daily basis, is off the charts. They ride on the top of the wave all day long. I surmise that their adrenalin levels remain extraordinarily high throughout the day. My guess is that all healthcare professionals must suffer from a severe case of PTSD. It amazes me that many more physicians aren't addicts or serial killers or haven't been committed to psych facilities.

It also amazes me that they don't simple keel over and die at a young age from stress and exhaustion.

Years ago, I was taking care of a critical patient. She was elderly and teetering on life vs death. The doctor assigned to her, had a reputation of being rude and condescending to the staff when he was under pressure. Bear in mind that he worked in a busy ER with me. Also note that everyone handles stress in a different way.

Algebra: High pressure ER + a doctor who crumbles under pressure= A riddled with PTSD, rotten egg doctor. In short, he was a physician with a bad attitude. His stress reliever was yelling and berating the staff members.

I remember thinking, "Uh oooo. Hopefully, Mrs. Elderly will not deteriorate because I am in NO MOOD to have to deal with Dr. Rotten Egg."

Of course, Mrs. Elderly stopped breathing, and so life saving measures were initiated. I called overhead for Dr. Rotten to please come immediately to room 28.

To my surprise, in walked Dr. Rotten Egg's alternate personality, or so it seemed. In this extraordinarily stressful situation, Dr. Egg politely asked for an update on this patient, which I gave him. He began to conduct this code situation in a very professional manner. Dr. Rotten Egg gave clear orders, remained calm, asked the staff in the room for any treatment suggestions, explained the plan of care for the next few minutes, and encouraged questions. Although this patient did not survive, Dr. Rotten Egg turned into Dr. Eggs Benedict.

He'd run the code perfectly and calmly and thoroughly without a tantrum of any sort. I was amazed. Had he taken up tennis or racquetball? Had he started psych meds?

I knew that I had to give him feedback so that his behavior at the code would be routine and not an exception.

After the patient was pronounced dead, I jetted to the Dr.'s office and asked Dr. Eggs Benedict for a few minutes of his time. I told Dr. Benedict that in my opinion, the code was perfectly run by him. I extolled all the great things he had done during that emergent and stressful ordeal. I expressed my gratitude for his calm, kind, and professional behavior. I told Dr. Benedict that I was planning on writing a letter to his boss about how well he had run the code.

I sent a lovely letter to the Chief of Staff and cc'd a copy to Dr. Eggs Benedict.

Dr. Benedict met me in the hallway a few days later. He had tears in his eyes. Apparently, Dr. Benedict had just been reprimanded for his poor behavior, a day prior to the code incident. He hugged me, thanked me, and told me that he appreciated my feedback.

I never again heard of anyone having an issue with Dr. B.

It was a life-changing event in my career. I finally got it. The lightbulb had come on. How the heck do doctors survive the routine stress without going bonkers? Don't get me wrong: I don't condone bad behavior. Taking frustrations out on someone else is unacceptable. But what should be done to help healthcare professionals deal with the insane amount of stress? Should routine psychiatric care be mandatory? Should an outlet like a free gym membership be a benefit of employment?

Again, I am amazed, looking back, that more doctors hadn't fallen to the floor, yelled and screamed, and thrown a tantrum. The daily pressure can send anyone off the bridge.

Physicians are a very special breed. Some are born knowing exactly why they arrived on this planet. Some realize their destiny over time. Some don't realize the immensity of their calling until their career is underway.

How doctors arrive at their medical career, is irrelevant. What is important is that they've signed up for an altruistic, lifelong state of mind, of service, and of being. They've agreed to care for humans at that human's lowest point in time. They've taken an oath to "do no harm." No pressure there!

Stories about these Superheroes flood into my brain as I compose this serious and emotional chapter in my book:

I have watched many doctors make the agonizing decision to cease CPR, after hours of attempting to save a life. These same physicians are expected, five minutes after a code ends, to see their next patient cheerfully and without missing a beat. They are expected to act like nothing tragic has just occurred. There is no chance to grieve or process the death they've just witnessed and actually commanded, especially after life-saving measures had failed.

I have seen patients arrive in the hospital feeling sick, worn down, or listless, and after hours or days of care from the medical team, led by doctors, they've left renewed and cured.

I have witnessed the abundance of compassion and sensitivity that physicians have shown patients and their families. Would you want to be the one to tell a mother that her child had died. Would you want to tell ANYONE that they have metastatic cancer or any fatal illness, for that matter? Would you want to let a father know that his son had just died in surgery?

Well, let me be very clear on this: Doctors are forced into the insurmountable task of delivering this kind of bad news. There is no other option. Either they go tell the family the news or no one does. Is there anything more stressful than that job?

I am not referring to just any bad news, like your car needs a new water pump, or your kid got a "C" in reading. I am referring to horrific, terrible news that no one wants to hear. I am talking about gut-wrenching, miserable info. These super humans are the messengers of all good and bad medical info.

Now go ahead and wipe off the tears from your face, because there are definitely wonderful things that doctors get to do, as well. I have seen them and witnessed the many happy endings in the world of healthcare.

To name just a few:

I have seen a doctor deliver a healthy baby emergently, in the ER, and proudly hold that cheezit up for the parents to see.

I have witnessed doctors giving critically-ill patients the news that they are on the mend.

I am blessed to have seen doctors telling many families that we were able to save the life of their loved ones.

I have even had the immense feeling of relief when a surgeon declared that my own relative did not have cancer.

Being a physician is not a job for a weak, selfish, or uncaring human. On the contrary. It is a profession that requires superpowers: a strong sense of leadership, a kind and gentle soul, some thoughtful communication skills, an intelligent and brilliant mind, a giver of the greatest kind, and an outer shell as strong as titanium.

Yes. Doctors ARE Superheroes. …so simply thanking them does NOT seem like enough!

What Do You Actually Do, Besides Give Out Pills?

My brother flew F4's out of Mather AFB in Sacramento, California, years ago. However, I never got a clear description of what he did in the Air Force after flying jets. It was usually too involved for civilians to understand.

Similarly, what an RN does would take days to explain. If we had to write down what we actually do as a nurse, we would need one large pack or 150 sheets of lined notebook paper to complete that task.

As non-medical humans who watched medical shows in the 1960s, 1970s, and 1980s may believe, we don't just give out pills.

Nursing administration has attempted to record our job description but has sorely missed at least ½ of what we really do. Here is just a tiny sampling of jobs that I did and personally feel should be added to our job description:

-Babysitting children (while the young mother leaves the room to speak with a physician about her husband, who was just diagnosed with brain cancer).

-Clean vomit, poop, and blood off the walls, floor, bed, etc. because the three housekeepers, who were hired to clean the entire facility, could not make it to the patient's room for hours.

-Spend hours upon hours on the phone with lab, x-ray, CT scan, MRI, treadmill, etc., in an effort to expedite patient care, or actually get them care.

-Spend hours trying to figure out how to work new equipment that was dropped onto the unit by aliens without any in-service or warning.

-Get coughed on, pooped on, sneezed on, vomited on, and bled on.

-Get slugged by a patient or family member, at any time, for no apparent reason.

-Feel guilty when we have to pee pee at work because there is always something that needs to be completed immediately.

-Perform the same responsibilities of a waitress (Listed under nursing skills).

-Spend a gazillion hours on hold, waiting to give report about a patient, to a different unit in the hospital, a different hospital, a nursing home, a police department, etc.

-Be guilted into skipping breaks due to "not enough staff."

-Feeling even more guilt when we have the flu, are hemorrhaging to death, or are taking our last breath because administration will imply that we are "abandoning the other staff members and humanity in general."

-Be verbally abused by most of the free world. (Al-Anon is available. Contact them for meetings, dates, and times.)

-Not be allowed to spend more than 10 minutes grieving over the death of another human being, because the other patients are waiting for us.

-Miss out on many holidays and weekends with family because the rest of the world "needs us more."

-Be required to lift, push, pull, and reposition patients as needed, even though the patient may weigh over 300 pounds, and you are 5'2" and weigh 120 pounds. There is no other human to help us on the hospital planet.

I could keep going with that list of jobs that nurses don't get credit for in the nursing job description. I just referenced a few that I dealt with and, for some reason, remembered. I know that you nurses have a bunch of your own.

In reality, a nursing job description usually includes, in some form, these topics:

-Conduct an individualized patient assessment on each of your assigned patients.

-Create a plan of care with the healthcare team.

-Conduct ongoing assessments and modify the plan of care, as needed.

-Perform therapeutic nursing interventions for each individual patient, as needed.

-Document patient assessments, plan of care, interventions, education, and patient responses to the care provided.

-Maintain confidentiality.

-Document some more.

-Maintain nursing skills competencies.

-Administer treatments as ordered.

-Document again.

-Administer medications to patients. Monitor the patient for medication effectiveness, side effects, and reactions.

-Promote a patient's health by completing the nursing process.

-Establish rapport with patients and their families.

-Assure quality of care by adhering to standards. Measure outcomes against patient care goals and hospital and regulatory standards.

-Maintain a safe working environment.

-Adhere to infection control policies.

-Document one more time.

-Maintain a relationship with the healthcare team by communicating patient information and participating in the plan of care as it evolves.

Do you get the idea? Nothing too detailed.

On the other hand, the list of recorded nursing skills is extensive, vast, and virtually endless. Here are just a few items on that list:

Draw venous blood.

Provide IV therapy, including, but not limited to, IV fluids and antibiotics.

Insert a urinary catheter and maintain it.

Insert a nasogastric tube and lavage; as needed.

Give all IV, IM, Sub Q, oral, nasal, etc. meds. as ordered.

Take and record vital signs per protocol.

Bathe, feed, and dress patients, as needed.

Evaluate all diagnostic test results and report abnormalities.

Dress wounds.

Aid doctors in procedures.

Educate patient on medical topics including diabetes, COPD, wound care, etc.

Provide tracheostomy care and suctioning as needed.

Administer and monitor procedural sedation.

Maintain all drains and tubes.

Help with critical decision-making.

Provide respiratory therapy treatments.

Assist with intubation.

Perform CPR.

Administer code medications.

Maintain seizure precautions.

Collect specimens to include urine, sputum and wounds.

Provide care to burn patients.

Use hypo/hyperthermia blankets appropriately.

Monitor and assess intake and output.

Use a central line or a PICC line per protocol.

Obtain blood gases.

Obtain blood cultures.

Plus, waitressing skills: clean bedside tables, wash yuck off of floors, as needed, obtain food from the cafeteria per patient's request, heat food as needed, and ask patients if they would like water, etc.

I am just touching the tip of the iceberg with that list of nursing skills. Plus, nurses do so much more than is ever recorded or recognized or mentioned.

I, for example, have cut the toenails of several elderly, neglected humans, before those nails curled into their flesh.

I have trimmed patients' pubic hairs, which were covered in poop and longer than the hair on the top of my head.

I have scrubbed and scrubbed dried dirt, worms and poop off of a man who was found on the ground, on his property, after a fall. He had been lying there for four or five days.

I have brushed the teeth of countless humans who were unable to do it for themselves for, what looked like, years.

I have shampooed blood and dirt off the hair of many, many accident victims.

In short, all nurses have similar stories of things that we have done, that are not listed in our job description. Like many professions, you never really fully know what your job entails until you live and work in that environment on a daily basis. I definitely did not even remotely know what I would be doing as an RN. I didn't know what I didn't know. NOW, I KNOW.

Suppose any human, who wanted to be a nurse, gets ahold of an accurate, thorough, and honest nursing job description, along with the encyclopedia of required nursing skills. In that case, they may rethink their career choice. These days, I surmise that the nursing profession might possibly die out, or at least have severe recruiting issues.

If Stress Kills, Nurses Have No Chance of Survival

Today, I asked Google what the top 10 most stressful jobs are in the USA. Not surprisingly, acute care nurses made the list.

I have always contended that you never understand how sick you actually are, until you have recovered.

Similarly, now that I have retired, I realize how sick I was for a few years. That illness that invaded my mind, body, and soul was called STRESS.

That chronic illness, caused by living in the nursing profession and working in the ER, day after day, is finally gone. Boy, was I sick for years? I now feel healthy, happy, and alive again.

Don't get me wrong. My nursing career was fantastic. I really didn't feel completely overwhelmed by stress until the year 2020.

During the Covid pandemic fiasco, I cried for six months, every day, driving home from work. The stress was insurmountable. Not only was there the usual immense stress from doing my nursing job in a busy ER, but added to that was a lack of protective supplies, a lack of help with patient care, and a lack of administration support. Nurses started leaving the profession in droves. For the first time in my career, I was unable to provide the high level, standard of care to my patients, that I was used to doing for many years.

The media, day after day, dispensed false info about what hospitals and medical personnel were dealing with. Daily (at least it felt like that), practices in the hospital changed. This led to chaos at my job. It was hard to keep up with the ever-changing opinions and so-called facts. I know this to be true because I lived it.

Just before I retired, I looked in the mirror at an unrecognizable human being. Who was that sick-looking person? Did she evolve into that unhealthy woman, simply by living in her career? How long would she last before she keeled over?

I was fatter than I had ever been. I was not, by any means obese, but I was carrying too much weight.

My dietary history was filled with only healthy eating, until a few years earlier. Stress had caused changes in my diet. I am guessing that my cortisol levels were higher than ever before.

I started work at 6:45 A.M. I would skip breakfast because I couldn't seem to get my stomach to want food before 9:00 A.M. My first food of the day was during my lunch break. The rest of my diet at work came from eating the ever-present junk food, scattered around the ER, which I mindlessly consumed.

When I got home from work, I would open the refrigerator and start eating anything and everything in sight, until I felt full. I was too tired to make a meal for myself at 4:00 P.M.

I had dark circles under my eyes. I had a permanent frown glued to my face. My posture looked poor. I was not sleeping well. I felt exhausted 24/7.

I looked terrible and I felt terrible. I was the poster child for burn out.

I love the people who preach "burn out prevention." They try to guide you into peace. Bless their hearts. They encourage travel, hobbies, meditation, etc.

Guess what. I was doing all of those things. I played piano and guitar. I was creating items with clay and even opened my own little pottery business (Robin Dainty Pottery). I traveled. I was meditating before bedtime. I would exercise by walking around the hospital during my lunch break. I was definitely trying to reduce my stress, but nothing was working. I was at the point of no return. I was burned out. I was Burned Out. I WAS BURNED OUT!

My usual, happy, fun attitude at work had turned into feelings of frustration, disappointment, sadness, and anger.

Nursing was no longer the career that I had loved so dearly. I didn't recognize my profession. The medical universe had drastically changed- and definitely NOT for the better.

My opinion: Within a few years, the healthcare system had deteriorated. Nursing practice took a nose dive. In the past, the central theme of my nursing job was to advocate for patients. We had the time to teach patients and answer questions, follow up with their test results, lend a listening ear, expedite care, etc.

I would introduce myself to each patient with the following:

"Hello. My name is Robin, like the bird. I am your nurse. I will be taking care of you today. I will be your advocate."

Suddenly, the theme of healthcare had changed. It felt like it happened over night. Medicine became BIG BUSINESS. Hospitals were publicizing their profits. (When did healthcare's focus become about money and not a patient's well-being?)

My opinion again: Healthcare went from a "patient wellness" theme to a "get them in and get them out," focus, the all-mighty dollar being the driving factor (Similar to an assembly line/factory). I didn't belong on the healthcare planet any longer. I dreamed of taking the first spaceship to another universe where I could take care of my patients as if they were my family, like I had always done.

Here I was, in a profession that defined me. I had always felt that I would work in nursing until I either died or couldn't walk anymore. I had loved my job for almost 40 years. But it wasn't the same job any longer.

I went on a girl's trip to Florida, surrounded by my posse. I spent hours talking to my dear sister-friends. One of these sisters we shall call Snow White, for she is lovely on the inside and out.

Snow is also a nurse, yet younger than me. She had left the ER several years earlier for the PACU (post anesthesia care unit) after experiencing the same things that I was going through. Snow White patiently spent hours listening to me gripe, cry, and vent. She knew that this behavior was not who I was. I was always the funny and happy one in our group. Snow encouraged me to live my truth, and follow my dreams.
Gosh, I love her.

That was it. That was the final straw. I had support from family and friends to leave the dysfunctional relationship that my career had evolved into.

Time to exit; stage left.

I thought that I was going to feel depressed when I retired. I was not 100% sure that I was making the right decision.

I was leaving my work family. They had been my roommates for many years. I laughed with them, cried with them, and lived with these peeps.

I felt very close to many people who worked in the hospital with me. How could I leave them behind? (Fortunately, many of my work family members are still part of my life.)

I was comforted by the thought that I could always find work as an RN if I hated retirement.

I loved my profession of nursing for soooo long. It was part of me. It defined me. But it was time to go.

I am happy to report that for the first three months after retirement, I would wake up at 5:00 A.M. with a smile on my face and yell "Weeeee!"

I would climb into my car, on the way to the gym at 7:00 A.M., and scream "Yeahhhhh," as loud as I could, for a full five seconds. It felt like I had hit the lotto. I was alive again.

Ahhhh. Freedom. Peace. It felt like a 50-pound weight had fallen off of my shoulders.

A few years later, I am very happy to state loudly, that retirement is the greatest invention in the history of this planet. I worked hard. It was time to play. I deserved it.

Today, if I may say so myself, I look great. I have lost 22 pounds; I stand up straight; and am able to smile again. I have plenty of time to do the things that I enjoy like creating pottery, playing music, travelling the world, and writing a book! Life just keeps getting better and better.

I am 100% certain that if you are a nurse reading this chapter, you can commiserate. I am certain that you and I come from the same mold and have survived the same very tough career.

Just know that being a nurse is wonderful, but there is life after our job. It is a beautiful life. It is a blank canvas, and we get to be the artist. We can paint the life that we have patiently waited to live.

If there is even a remote chance that you can retire early, may I suggest that you do it? I contacted a financial advisor who assured me that the time was right.

A financial advisor will go over your "intake and output" (your assets and liabilities) and advise you accordingly about the right time to say good-bye to nursing.

Like Florence Nightingale, most nurses spend their lives devoted to caring for the sick and injured. It is one of the most unselfish professions. But, at some point, we all need to take care of ourselves before our expiration date.

The only thing stopping you from the life you want, is YOU!

Now on to a story. This single event in my life, helped me realize that we all have different definitions of stress. Also, we all deal with stress differently and it affects us differently.

This real-life tale happened during my tenth year of practicing nursing.

It went pretty close to this:

I was living with a lovely roommate in the Bay area of Northern California. We shall call this roommate Elaine, after the character in the TV show **Seinfeld**.

Elaine was a manager at a popular clothing chain. She loved her job and took pride in the success of this particular store.

I was working in a busy ER. A baby, with congenital issues, had passed away on this day. The medical staff desperately tried, for hours, to save her. Unfortunately, to no avail. The parents cried and cried. The stress and sadness overtook everyone in the emergency room.

I didn't even remember my drive back to my apartment, that day. I headed up to my living quarters in the elevator, walked inside, and fell onto the couch sobbing. I stayed there for a long time, reliving the events of the day and wondering if we could have done anything differently.

At approximately 9:00 P.M., the door to our apartment opened abruptly and slammed shut. In walked Elaine, tossing her purse onto our little round dining room table.

Me: Startled. I sat up straight on the couch and asked, "Everything ok?"

Elaine: "No. I had a horrible day. I am stressed to the max."

Me: "What's wrong. What happened?"

Elaine: Frantically walking around our tiny kitchen and dining room: "I have to start getting ready for the Christmas holiday. I just got a huge clothing shipment in. I don't know where I am going to store ½ of the boxes. I never planned to get this much inventory."

"I have to make some major decisions by tomorrow. I don't know whether to put the red holiday clothing in the showcase or the green ones. Do I put the red clothes close to the entrance to the store? Should I mix the colors up and scatter them around the store? This stress is going to kill me."

Me: I didn't respond. I couldn't think of a thing to say. I just stared at her.

How could Elaine be freaking out over clothes?

A lightbulb came on in my brain. Like a bolt of lightning, I finally got clarity.

I realized at that moment that Elaine and I were existing on two completely different planets. We were walking down different roads in life. Elaine would never be able to comprehend the stress that I endured on this day, unless she worked as a nurse in a busy ER. I didn't understand her stressing out over the location of clothes. Again, you have to live in it to get it.

I never divulged to Elaine, the horrible day that I had and still relive periodically. No need.

All I know is that after this experience, I realized that nurses are some of the toughest, most resilient super heroes on this planet!

Nurses Are a Different Breed of Animal

Under the title "Human Race," nurses should be further differentiated into a category all by ourselves. My guess is that nurses are probably born under the human race category, but within a year or two of working in the nursing profession, they should be abruptly reclassified. We just don't fit the mold of average homo sapiens.

Please allow me some liberties in this chapter. When I say "we," I mean the nurses who I have worked with, have come in contact with, who have been in my circle, etc. We all are made out of the same mold.

Nurses are a unique breed among humanity. We may look like everyone else, but we are not even close to others in how we think or act, especially in a crisis. I will speak for most nurses when I declare that we don't understand people's overreaction to minor mishaps, or major ones for that matter. Nurses believe that there is no need to freak out over any situation. Life is too short for that.

If you have worked as a nurse in a hospital, you have seen an exorbitant amount of death, trauma, and injuries. You have been on the battlefield, fighting sickness of all sorts, ever since you graduated nursing school. Years and years of living in a war zone can take its toll. I will bet the farm, that all of us nurses could get that PTSD diagnosis.

I will go out on a limb and speak for my sister and brother nurses when I say that we all feel spiritually blessed to still be alive on this planet. We have seen too much. We have felt too much. And we definitely know too much about how fragile life is and how valuable our time on earth is. We refuse to sweat the small stuff.

We act differently. We think differently. We respond differently than most humans to most situations.

Here are a few examples from my list of how we think and act as nurses:

-We all hate working when there is a full moon. It's true. Weird things happen when that white globe in the sky shines brightly. Volumes of odd humans flock to the hospital, with weird complaints.

-We will get upset if anyone at work says "It sure is quiet around here." That statement brings about the worst day in months.

-We believe that a new law should be passed that requires a permit to reproduce. We have seen some horrible parenting which includes abuse and neglect. (I definitely take better care of my dogs than some humans take care of their children.) I firmly believe that in order to be a parent, you should have to go to parenting school and take exams.

-We believe that "stupidity" should be a diagnosis. Common sense does not live in everyone.

-We don't get upset when a patient wants to leave abruptly. As I have said to many humans who were threatening to leave the hospital, "This is not a prison. You are free to come and go as you wish." …except for psych patients on a 5150 hold.

-People often forget that they are not the only ones requiring care in the hospital. Lunch is low on the priority list, in the ER. It comes after a heart attack patient, a hemorrhaging patient, and pretty much all patient diagnoses. If a patient is hungry, then nurses agree that they can't be that sick. They can wait for the grub.

-We don't miss a beat. While eating a meal, we can discuss blood and guts in front of non-medical family and friends. We forget that it is a disgusting habit because we do it at work, all the time. Sorry.

-We are diagnosing medical history on everyone we see at the grocery store, bank, restaurant, amusement park, or anywhere, for that matter. I have predicted the medical future of a family friend and been spot on. (Gosh, Robin, get a life.)

-We check the veins out of people in front of us, in lines. We justify this odd habit by telling ourselves we need this info in case the person collapses and needs an IV. That is not really true. It is just a habit. We are always checking veins on our new patients at work. This habit obviously carries on into our community.

-We attempt to predict an intoxicated patient's actual blood alcohol level. It's fun. It's a game. Come on people. We need at least a crumb to keep our spirits up.

-We desire to present a daily award for the best actor/actress patient in a dramatic role.

For example, some patients arrive yelling and screaming in pain while eating a burrito or chatting on the phone. I assume the behavior is for a dramatic effect. (I, personally, wanted to sculpt a penis shaped trophy out of clay to give out.) I forgot to put that idea into the suggestion box. Drats.

-We absolutely ignore humans who are pierced and tattooed all over their bodies, yet complain vehemently about getting an injection or IV. How is it that one chooses to have a zillion little needles stuck into them over hours and hours of time, but they insist on giving me grief over a needle stick that lasts 0.01 of a second. That boggles my mind.

-We lose pens faster than Pilot can make them. On the flip side, we take pens from any business willing to give them out. With the advent of computers, we rarely need a pen today. At work, our minds are on more important things. We pretty much could care less about pens, except when we need one. At that point, we would offer to buy anyone, coffee or donuts, in order to get one.

-We will never, ever say or think, "It can't get any worse," because we are 100% sure, that just by saying or thinking it, it will get much worse.

-As a nurse, I have definitely seen more private parts than most humans, including all the prostitutes in Texas. No offense, but seeing a naked body does not affect me, or most nurses, at all. It just proves that getting "turned on" is 100% mentally motivated. Clean up and wear a suit and all bets are off.

-We can sit or stand anywhere and eat. We can consume a five-course dinner in under two minutes. There are sick people out there. The guilt won't let us relax and chew our food. We pretty much inhale food and snacks.

-We can lie down anywhere, including on the floor, on the bench seat in the breakroom, on an empty patient bed, on the grass near the medical office building, on the concrete walkway by the cafeteria, and sleep there, from sheer exhaustion. I can power nap in 15 minutes and feel like I had seven to eight hours of sleep. I once worked seven double shifts in seven days straight. That's right: 16 hours a day for 7 days. I was much younger, so sleep was not that important. My dinner was spent sleeping on the table in the break room. Exhaustion finally won out.

-We think that eating any food out of a bedpan or emesis basin is normal. In fact, we can drink water out of a urinal. You have to do what you have to do when no cups or bowls are available in your general vicinity. Truth.

Those are just the ones that come to my mind today. The list is endless.

Our nursing behaviors probably seem heartless, cold, mean, uncaring and definitely weird and bizarre. Well, maybe they are. You try living in the world of a nurse on a daily basis, year after year. You will either develop coping skills or crumble. The coping skills are less harmful, for sure.

For 13 years of my career, I worked inside a hospital. (The ER and clinics are considered outside of the hospital.) I was different then. People who were admitted for surgery, cancer, heart attacks, etc., needed to be hospitalized. They needed my help. They were sick. They were kind and appreciative. I was sympathetic to their needs.

When I transferred to ER in 1995, I was aghast at the staff's behaviors. They appeared uncaring, intolerant, and unsympathetic. I did not understand why those ER nurses acted that way until I lived it.

ER nurses are different from all other nurses. The volumes of rude, ignorant, entitled, mean, unappreciative humans who flood into the ER daily, with ridiculous complaints, would make ANYONE beg to be transported to a new planet. It didn't take long for me to see humanity at its worst. It only took a few years for me to develop coping skills in order to survive other people's behaviors.

Whenever an ER patient would become abusive, I would lower my voice and let them know that "I was not getting paid to be abused." They would no longer have the privilege of having me give them great care. I would then leave the room. I would immediately report the patient's behavior to my charge nurse and ask for a different assignment.

The majority of the time, within an hour of the conflict, Mr. Rude patient would request that I return to the room so that he could apologize. Mr. Rude would request that I resume taking care of him.

The other few abusive patients who never apologized included a meth addict who screamed at me and wanted to speak to the head of the hospital because I woke her up by taking her vital signs and giving her breakfast at 9:00 A.M., and a morbidly obese woman who resented my request to have her assist me with sitting her bootie up at the bedside.

My point is, ER staff members are at the forefront of some very insane and unacceptable behaviors and verbiage. The result is that ER nurses have developed a force field around us. That layer is made of kryptonite, titanium, or diamonds, which are the hardest, naturally-occurring substances on earth. (I wish. That would certainly bring more value to our profession.) This force field or wall is an absolute necessity. It has to be around us, or we couldn't/wouldn't work in the ER. This wall protects the patient from our responses. It protects us from being fired.

The wall has arms. It places duct tape over our mouths when we are about to say what we really want to say.

Without that wall, we would "go off." There would be nothing but yelling, screaming, and fighting between staff and patients. The police would be called. There would be mayhem. This is MY THEORY anyway.

The staff that I worked with, heard me say, the following on many occasions: "On my last day of nursing here in the ER, I am going to say exactly what comes to my mind. I won't hold anything back."

My peeps all said that they wanted to witness me on my final day.

Unfortunately, I never got my wish. My last day of work was spent tearfully saying adios to all of the wonderful staff members around the hospital, who I'd worked with for many years. (Much heathier than what I had envisioned.)

Here are just a few situations that have frequently put my force field and mouth to a test:

1. People who entered the ER with "severe abdominal pain" eating Doritos and a Burger King Whopper, but insisted on being seen immediately.

(How would you respond?)

2. People who just arrived in an ambulance to the ER, who immediately stated, "I am hungry. When is dinner served?"

(I usually responded to that statement with, "Let's get you feeling better so that you can jet to one of the 10 restaurants that surround this wonderful facility." Not what I really wanted to say.)

3. People who arrived at the ER with a few minutes of nausea as their only symptom and concern.

(1/2 the world has a bit of nausea daily. Just watching the news gives me nausea. On my planet, these humans are redirected.)

4. People who had the worst headache of their lives, but were able to read a magazine, go outside and smoke a cigarette, and yell at me for the wait times.

(Like I have control of anything in the ER, let alone wait times. If I did, trust me, things would be very different.)

5. People who came to the ER, with minor complaints, who had a doctor's appointment "in an hour." They wanted to be seen faster. They had things to do.

(…and this is why ERs are constipated.)

6. People who arrived in the ER, having NO CLUE as to what medications they took on a routine basis. When asked for a medication list, they respond with, "Two pinks, a blue and a yellow."

(The number of times I had to explain why this was an issue, far exceeds the number of humans living in Sacramento, California.)

7. People who came to the ER for a toothache that they had for a month, but never thought to call a dentist.

(Either I ramble on about this issue or continue on…)

8. People who were tattooed, pierced, and smoked cigarettes and marijuana but had no $ for Tylenol for a headache.

(Either I ramble on about this issue or continue on…)

9. People who told me their diagnosis and treatment plan before I even introduced myself. They used Dr. Google.

(Why don't you let us do our job? When we are all done, you can let us know if this second opinion was spot on or not. Guess we don't need medical professionals anymore. The world has Dr. Google.)

10. People who asked the triage nurse when they would be able to see an ER doctor.

(Note: After triage, those humans who have never watched the news, been to an ER in the last 10 years, or have any medical peeps in their family, neighborhood, or circle, should receive a handout which states, "We see the most critical patients first. Thus, we cannot give you an appointment time. Unless of course, you can see into the future and tell us the severity of each patient entering the ER today.")

11. People who answered a nurse's questions with, "It's in my chart."

(That's nice. Please give me one full day to read through your chart which could be as long as a Steinbeck novel. Or, you can opt just to answer the question. Jeeeeezzzz.)

12. People who brought their entire family with them to an overcrowded ER.

(I already rambled on about this issue in a previous chapter.)

13. People who didn't answer any question you asked without giving you a 10-minute dissertation.

(We need simple answers in the ER. We have no time for anything else. I would love to stay and chat, but my other critical ER patients may get mad.)

14. People who insisted on telling nurses and doctors how to do their job.

(Oh boy. I better stop here. Hopefully, you get the idea.)

In my opinion, nurses have immeasurable amounts of restraint, composure, patience, and obvious self-control, plus a very strong force field and extra strong duct tape. Otherwise, nurses would all end up in jail.

The Medal of Honor is the highest military decoration awarded by Congress to a member of the armed services for gallantry and bravery in combat at the risk of life above and beyond the call of duty.

Hopefully you agree that a nurse deserves The Medal of Honor, upon retirement, for surviving years and years of gallantry and bravery in unimaginable combat.

Precepting or Training Camp

Both of my parents taught school during their lives. They wanted me to be a teacher as well. My grandfather was a teacher. My sisters were teachers. My brother is now a teacher. But I swore that I would never want to do that job.

I know my limitations. I know that I could never tolerate rude kids or their parents. I would blow a gasket in dealing with spoiled children. I don't have diplomacy built into my make-up. I had no idea that nursing would test my resolve as much as teaching would have.

My unwillingness to enter into a teaching career backfired. I fought against being an educator during my younger years. I entered teaching through a back door.

After nursing school, I immediately began to precept new hires. I was eventually asked to teach a clinical class for first-semester nursing students. I agreed to do so. I am not sure why. When I look back, instructing nursing students and registered nurses on how to deliver superior care didn't fall under the teaching category in my brain. It fell under the teaching nurses to "treat others the way you want to be treated" category.

How did it happen? I swore that I would never be a teacher and before I knew it, I was the lead preceptor.

Funny how genetics works.

During my career, I trained a lot of healthcare professionals, from student nurses, EMT's, and paramedics, to new grads, new hire RNs and transfer nurses from other facilities. I would always tell them to ask questions. "No question is stupid," I preached. I assisted teaching in new graduate nursing programs in several different hospitals. By far, I trained more nurses and nursing students than any other staff members who I knew.

I am very happy to tell you that I had a part in many success stories. I was at ground zero for the training of nurses who are now hospital administrators, educators, charge nurses, flight nurses, staff nurses, clinic nurses, PACU nurses, GI nurses, etc. I feel like a proud grandparent.

I absolutely loved educating nurses. It was obviously in my blood. I had tried to fight the pull into education, but the universe had a different plan for me.

Looking back now, I am very happy to tell you that educating nurses filled up my heart and soul. I loved teaching. It was apparently my destiny.

I would call my nursing students, and new grads, "my puppies." It was an endearing term. I would explain to them that they were eager to learn like a two-month-old puppy. These new nurses and students would be with me for three to six months. I would provide them with a solid nurse training program so that they could take great care of me one day. After that time, they would hopefully know enough to go out on their own, provide excellent care, and be safe in the medical world. They would be equivalent to a one-year-old doggy in skills, behavior and hopefully attitude.

I encouraged them to ask questions. I would say, "You don't know what you don't know. You become dangerous if you think you know and don't ask questions before you act." Some of the students understood that phrase. Others had no clue what I meant, until they "fell on their face," or **someone** fell on **his** face.

Example:

I was concerned about a nursing student who I was precepting. She was in her last year of nursing school. Let's call her Brittany from the tv show **Glee**.

Brittany always looked like a deer staring at headlights. I had to frequently invite her into a patient's room. I would say, "Brittany, it is very hard to take care of your patient while standing in the hallway." Brittany would nod and come into the room, hesitantly. She was much more comfortable staring inside the room than actually entering the room.

On one very hot and sunny day, I asked Brittany to wheel a patient (Mr. Aged Man) out of the ER. I explained to Brittany that Mr. A.M.'s wife was going to retrieve her car and pull it up to the front of the emergency room. Brittany needed to assist the wife in getting Mr. Aged Man out of the wheelchair and into the car. That was the totality of her assignment.

Mr. Aged Man was approximately 89 years old, give or take a few years. He was steady on his feet, but a bit confused at times. Brittany stated that she understood the assignment. She had no questions.

After about five minutes of caring for a critical patient, I noted, that Brittany was standing in the hallway, staring at me, instead of standing outside with Mr. A.M. I walked out of the room and asked Brittany if Mr. Aged Man got into the car and left for home.

Brittany stared at me and responded, "I don't know."

I ran to the entrance of the ER and out the front door. There, I saw Mr. Aged Man, face down on the hot pavement. His wife had not arrived to pick him up, as of yet.

Do you think that Brittany followed me outside. No. Brittany, the deer, remained in the hallway.

After carefully assessing this patient and deeming him ok to be moved, I sat Mr. Aged up and assisted him back into the wheelchair. I wheeled Aged back into the ER and back into the room that he had just left. I assisted him into bed. He had multiple abrasions on his face, hands, and arms.

Brittany stood in the hallway, not offering any assistance, while watching the event unfold, as I wheeled Mr. Aged right by her. After getting him settled in bed and letting the charge nurse and an ER doctor as well as Mr. Aged's wife know what had happened, I instructed Brittany to head to the break room.

I arrived into the break room where Brittany sat at the table. I pulled up a chair and sat across the table from this deer.

Here is how that conversation went:

Me: "Brittany. Is everything ok with you today?"

Brittany: "Yes. What happened to Mr. Aged?"

Me: "He must have stood up from the wheelchair and fallen forward. Why did you leave Mr. Aged in the wheelchair before his wife arrived and before he'd gotten into his car? You know that he is confused at times, correct?"

Brittany: "Yes. I know that he can be confused. I guess that I didn't understand what you wanted me to do."

Me: "I asked you to wheel Mr. Aged out the front of the ER and assist Mr. Aged's wife in getting him into the car. You said that you understood the assignment, correct?"

Brittany: "Yes, but I really didn't understand exactly what you wanted me to do."

Me: "If you didn't understand what I wanted you to do, then why didn't you ask?"

Brittany: "I don't know. I guess that I thought his wife would be there soon enough to help him. I didn't want you to think that I was stupid."

Me: Thinking to myself: Too late. This story needs to be in the chapter entitled Ignorant or Uneducated.

Me: Let's try this a different way, I thought to myself: "Brittany, is there a reason you would think that I might declare you stupid for asking clarification on something that you didn't understand?"

Brittany: "I think that I am just scared of everything right now."

Me: "Brittany, no question is stupid. Not asking questions can result in harm. That is exactly what just happened. Remember when I explained to you that you don't know what you don't know and that the only remedy is to ask questions so that no one gets hurt?"

Brittany: "Oh yeah. I remember that. Will he be ok?"

Me: "Yes Brittany. He will be ok. Please let this be a lesson for you. The only way to clarify what needs to be done, is by asking questions. No question is stupid. Questions prevent injuries. Mr. Aged could have sustained much more serious injuries. Please, please ask questions and never ever abandon a confused human who might fall if left alone. Do you understand?

Brittany nodded.

I was still not convinced that Brittany understood the importance of asking questions.

Onward.

I would tell the nurses who I was precepting, that they would develop their own nursing practice over time, based on safety, efficiency, knowledge, nursing care standards, and a desire to take care of people exactly how they would want their family taken care of, providing they loved their family.

One absolutely lovely nurse, who I had trained years before, applied for a charge nurse position in the ER. We shall call her Elsa, as in the princess in **Frozen**, for she was and still is, beautiful, inside and out.

During the interview for the position, in front of administrators, she was asked something along the lines of who inspired her in her nursing practice.

Her answer was Robin Dainty. Me. Wow! What a compliment.

She stated that I taught her to treat every patient as if they were her family. Tears.

I would tell my students that my years as a nurse were considered continual research years, aimed at formulating the ever-changing, very best patient care practices.

Another nurse who I had precepted, told me this story about a brand-new nurse she was training. Let's call the experienced nurse Doggy and the new nurse, Puppy.

Puppy: "Why are you doing that procedure that way?"

Doggy: "Because Robin trained me on how to do it, and she has over 30 years of research."

Tears again.

My own research and the subsequent formulation of my own nursing practice, began immediately upon my graduation from nursing school.

Here is an example that happened to me early on in my nursing practice:

If my patient needed her hair shampooed, I would hunt for something called a shampoo board. It could take me 15 minutes to find that item on a busy hospital unit.

The shampoo board was a really uncomfortable, plastic, concave, two feet across, board, that would be placed under a patient's neck so that I could wash her hair. The water would flow into the concave reservoir and be directed out of one side into a garbage can.

One day, I saw an LVN/LPN walk into my patient's room with a plastic trash bag, three towels, three folded blankets and a urinal. I thought she was going to provide the patient with a urinal and change the bedding. I followed behind to help her with the task.

She put a plastic bag down on the upper portion of the bed. She placed the 3 blankets on top of the plastic bag. She had my patient lie down face up, with the 3 blankets being used as her pillow. Next, she tucked two towels around the patient's neck and chest and handed the patient the third towel to wipe her face as needed. She filled the urinal with warm water, wet the patient's hair and began the shampoo process. Afterward, she tossed the wet blankets and towels into the linen cart and the plastic bag into the garbage. Wow. How easy was that? It certainly was much more comfortable for the patient than that hard plastic shampoo board.

I instantly adopted that practice and used it forevermore.

After several years of "research" or nursing practice, my personal ways of doing things took shape. I watched other nurses, asked questions and noted what practices worked best for the patient. I kept in mind that quality care, nursing standards of care, as well as safety measures, were of utmost importance.

During a nurse's orientation, on day one, I would list all the reasons why nursing is the greatest profession on earth. I would explain to my student that when humans are at their worst, when a family member is dying, when a pandemic hits, no actors, politicians, athletes, or CEOs show up to be at the bedside to provide medical and emotional support. Nurses are on the front line of that war: battling disease, preventing death, and providing comfort to the sick and injured every single day. I would proudly claim that without nurses, humanity would have a very difficult time surviving on earth, for who would care for the sick?

Very, very proud nurse here.

On the flip side, I have a few stories that demonstrate why nursing is definitely not for everyone.

I was precepting the sweetest new graduate who looked like Cinderella. In fact, let's call her Cinderella.

Cinderella was scared and shy. I could tell that she felt this way during our initial conversation on her first day in a pre-post op/trauma unit. She followed me around for a few days and assisted with procedures.

On the third day of her training, it was her turn to take on her own nursing assignment. I gave her three of the six assigned patients, to care for. I took care of the other three.

All of our patients were elderly. I kept checking with her to see how she was doing. I gave her the easiest patients, so I thought.

To this day, I am not sure how this unfolded, but in the space of an eight-hour shift, all three of her patients died. Two of them were no codes. The other patient was a full code. He had passed away while taking a nap. The dietary help found him deceased when she went in to sit him up for dinner. He had been dead for at least an hour.

Three deaths in one eight-hour shift seem unbelievable to me now. This story happened in the mid-1980s.

Poor Cinderella. Upon the death of her third patient, she began to audible cry. I guided her to the nursing lounge and gave her the best pep talk that I could come up with under the circumstances. We both felt very sad. I felt terribly helpless.

Cinderella came to work fully dressed in street clothes the next day. She asked to speak with me privately.

Cinderella explained through tears, that her parents had made her go to nursing school. She had completed her Bachelor in Nursing only because her parents insisted that she do it. After the prior horrible night, Cinderella knew that nursing was definitely not for her.

Cinderella declared that she was going to apply to several airlines because she had always wanted to be a flight attendant.

I hugged her and wished her well. I assured her that nursing was not a career for everyone. I encouraged her to follow her dreams.

The next story involves a paramedic student. I was assigned to precept him during his final semester of classes. He needed something like 160 hours working in the ER to complete his paramedic program.

Let's call him Ivan. He was from the Ukraine.

Ivan was an attractive man in his late 20s. He carried himself with confidence. He initially seemed eager to learn.

On day one, I reviewed with Ivan my expectations, exactly how his time would be spent in the ER, and what he needed to do to pass the preceptorship. He said that he was eager to get started and complete the program.

After reviewing his calendar, he informed me of the days that he would be available to train with me in the ER.

During his first day, I noted him speaking with several security guards that he "knew from his church." I certainly did not mind him saying hello.

The problem arose on the second day of his preceptorship, when I noted that he was spending more time chatting with these gents, than taking care of his patients.

This issue continued onto his third training day. I addressed this problem with him. He claimed that he understood and would curtail the conversation with the guards.

As the second week of training started with Ivan, I noted his indifference to caring for his patients. He sat at the desk often, staring at his phone. Several times, I encouraged him to check on his patients, and, if nothing else, see if any other nurses needed assistance with things like IV starts. I felt like I had to keep prodding him to move.

The final straw happened during his third week of training. I had to insert a Foley catheter.

Me: "Ivan. Would you like to come and insert this urinary catheter into this patient? I will help you and talk you through it."

Ivan: "Not really. I don't have to do that as a paramedic."

Me: Wow. I was speechless for a second. "Ok. I am sure that there are many things that you will do here in the ER that you won't do out in the field.

Examples include looking at lab work, watching a treadmill test, seeing X-rays being done, etc. I am here to give you a foundation of learning. If you have that foundation, you will be able to explain to the patients who you are transporting, exactly what will be happening to them. You will be able to allay their fears. You will be able to answer questions with knowledge-based answers."

Ivan: Looking unimpressed. "Ok. I will do it, he hesitantly replied."

Me: I was disgusted.

As I retrieved the supplies, I wondered if I was doing the right thing by encouraging Ivan to do the procedure of inserting a Foley catheter. I decided to go ahead and try to guide him through the process.

I had to keep repeating each instruction for inserting the catheter.

Halfway through the procedure, more than unhappy with his lack of interest in what he was doing, I told Ivan to take his gloves off, wash his hands, and I would meet him at the nurse's station. I completed the procedure.

I walked out of the room, and went straight to Ivan, who was once again, sitting in a chair staring at his phone. I instructed Ivan to meet me in the supply room.

Here is how that conversation went:

Me: "Ivan, what's up?"

Ivan: "What do you mean?"

Me: "Since you arrived, I have not felt that you have any interest in learning anything here at the hospital. Am I wrong?"

Ivan: "I don't know."

Me: "Let me rephrase this. Does the thought of helping people crank your soul? Do you long to work in the medical profession? Ivan, do you want to be a paramedic?"

Ivan: "Wow. You are the first person to ask me that question."

Me: "That's sad."

Ivan: "No. No. I don't want to be a paramedic. I don't want to work in the medical field. It makes me sick to see things here. My parents made me take this course."

Me: "Ivan. I am sorry to hear your answer. Let's discuss this situation for a minute. First and foremost, you are deserving of a career that gets you excited to go to work. If medicine is not it, no harm, no foul. You tried it on, and it didn't fit you."

"The world is deserving of caregivers who care. If you have recognized that you don't belong in the paramedic profession before graduation, kudos to you."

"You need to find something that cranks your soul, Ivan. Colleges have career testing that can help you narrow your interests into career choices that would best suit you."

"Next, please don't waste any more of my time. Other students want to precept with me. Please don't waste any more of your time in a career that does not interest you."

"And last but not least, I wish you a wonderful life, Ivan."

Ivan had tears in his eyes as I spoke. He stood up and left immediately, without saying another word. He didn't even say goodbye.

I was gutted. Did I upset him? Was he angry at my rant? Should I have been gentler in my approach? I stayed awake that night, feeling awful.

The next day, I arrived at work. I was in the breakroom, waiting for my shift to start when I heard an overhead page. "Robin Dainty to the front of the ER. Now please." I got scared. Usually that meant a family member or friend had checked into the ER.

I quickly walked to the front, pressed the button to open the door from the ER to the waiting room, and there stood Ivan with a bunch of flowers in his hand. He ran up to me and gave me the biggest hug. He handed me a card and the flowers. Ivan stated, "You changed my life. I could never thank you enough. I will never forget you."

Now it was my turn to cry.

And So It Goes…

It has taken me months to figure out what to say in this final chapter. I don't want this book to end. I don't want the stories from my nursing career to stop flowing through my brain. I never want to forget them. I want to savor all of those memories forever and ever, because the good ones and the bad ones have taught me so much.

My history in nursing is filled with seemingly endless tales that overtake my thoughts throughout the day, in my sleep, while running errands, and when chatting with friends or family. Some of these memories can bring me to tears at the drop of a hat. (Is that the definition of PTSD?) Other stories make me feel like a superhero.

Nursing is exactly why I am on this planet. But, thank God, I am not alone, for many other humans have arrived here with the same destiny.

I always joke that in our next lives, we nurses will desire to be ignorant, wealthy, humans who care only about superficial things. Due to our stupidity, nothing will phase us. We will have the depth of a frog pond. Our biggest crisis will be breaking a nail on a Sunday. Our lives will revolve around planning our next European vacation and deciding which expensive restaurant will be serving our dinner. I believe that this will happen because we used up our "living in stress requirements" during this life and should get a free pass in the next one. Don't you agree?

However, nurses are by no means operating alone.

I have worked with not only stellar nurses, but also with amazing doctors, unit secretaries, techs, housekeepers, supply clerks, paramedics, EMT's, physical therapists, etc. "It takes a village" is an understatement. So many knowledgeable humans have worked their butts off to get patients to feel better. Many more medical peeps have done everything, even out of their job description, to save lives. People who work in the medical profession are superheroes, without a doubt, if I may say so myself.

Nursing is such a wonderful career, where people are allowed to practice medicine as I was able to for so many years.

I was able to provide superior care to humans at a low point in their lives. I had the time to educate people about their disease as well as teach them the best way to care for their illness.

I performed tests and had time to look up the results so that the doctor and I could figure out what to do next. I carried out orders which ultimately made patients feel better. I had time to feed patients, wash them, help them, and comfort them. I discharged people to safe and secure environments. And in my mind, for many years of my nursing career, we all lived happily ever after.

But something happened. Something drastically changed in just a few short years. Greed overtook healthcare.

The toxic changes that have occurred in this beautiful, selfless, caring, and honorable profession of nursing, make me vomit. Financial gain has destroyed the full intent of Florence Nightingale. She is probably rolling over in her grave.

If this doesn't make you angry, it should at least make you very, very sad.

But I don't want to end this book with sadness. I want to share with you the essence of nursing. I want to let you know what nurses are really about.

Joe Becigneul posted the following on Facebook Jan 29, 2022:

Joe wrote, "I want to pass this on. I did not write it, but it is worthy of a moment of your time."

"We feel this in our bones":

"ER/Critical Care/Healthcare workers are a different kind of creature."

"We condition ourselves to roll with the punches…no matter how brutal…you roll. Somebody's life depends on it."

"Our eyes see the unfathomable…sights that would keep a normal person awake at night…but we roll."

"We condition ourselves to not feel it…not take life too seriously…we know how fragile and brief it is…we are reminded every time we swipe that time clock…every time…and we roll."

"I picked a lady up off the floor this evening after she walked out of the room where her husband died. She dropped to her knees…she wailed…she cried out for the father of her children…and without batting an eye, I knelt beside her and helped her the best way I could…death had won again."

"We become numb…our hearts don't feel things like the hearts who are protected from this type of consistent and repeated defeat…we cope…and maybe too well."

"Maybe we come off as cold and emotionally unavailable. Maybe we aren't approachable."

"We come off a little bossy…because we have to be good patient advocates…to be the person our patient needs."

"Be patient with the ER/ICU nurse/RTs/EMS/PD/FD in your life. Your eyes have not seen what theirs have."

"You haven't felt it…you haven't battled death as much and as hard as they have."

"You could never see their world through their eyes…because if they love you…they wouldn't want you to…they will protect you from it."

"Healthcare PTSD is at an all-time high, but your family member would never expose you to that. Be patient and kind with your ER/CC nurse/RT…you never know what battlefield they just walked off of."

"With love,

A tired, drained, yet passionate healthcare worker.

That prose touched me deeply. I wanted to share it with you."

What I want you to take from this book is that nurses have many wonderful qualities that spill over into how they care for humanity:

We represent a selfless spirit:

-We work long hours and overtime, and we often miss holidays with our families and friends.

We are the definition of emotionally strong:

-We hold a woman who we just met, while she cries over the sudden loss of her husband. We help to resuscitate a young person who overdosed.

We are kind:

-We assist people to the bathroom. We clean up vomit and poop on people that we have never met before. We brush a patient's teeth when he can't do it himself.

We are thoughtful:

-We make sure that patients are not discharged before they are ready to go home. We make sure that their food is heated up and not cold. We change their pillow cases because we notice there is blood on their linen.

We are brutally truthful:

-We let patients know what is happening and what to expect. We answer questions and provided information, even if it evokes sadness.

We are advocates:

-We speak up for quality care for our patients. We let the healthcare team know what patients want and need.

We are intelligent:

-We keep up with the ever-changing, patient-care protocols.

We care:

-If we didn't care, we would have chosen a different profession.

This list could go on for pages. I will stop it here because I think you get the idea that nurses are incredible human beings who care for, and advocate for, others. I am proud to be one of them.

Here is a final story. It happened to me. It exemplifies the passion that I had for my job as a nurse. It is about advocating for what is best for patients and treating all of them as if they were family members. It is a story of hope and kindness. I am confident that all nurses have stories similar to this one:

I was approximately 35-years-old, working in a teaching hospital in Northern California. I was a charge nurse on a step-down unit working 6:45 A.M.-3:15 P.M.

(A step-down unit contains patients who are less critical than ICU patients but who are more critical than med-surg patients.) As a busy section of the hospital, this unit was always filled with critical patients. Many of these patients were on ventilators, or had new tracheostomies, or had critical IV medications being infused.

One afternoon, a man arrived to the step-down unit with critical symptoms. He was an engineer who was approximately 55-years-old. Let's call this patient Andy Dufresne from my favorite all-time movie, **Shawshank Redemption**.

The patient, Andy, was a kind, intelligent, and caring man, who had been dealt an unfair hand, just like the lead character in **Shawshank**. He was quickly diagnosed in the ER with Guillain-Barre, a rare illness in which the immune system attacks the nerves. A bacterial or viral infection can trigger it.

Andy came to the ER with complaints of weakness and tingling of his hands and feet. The symptoms can progress quickly, and that is exactly what was happening to Andy.

He arrived on the step-down unit and immediately became short of breath. Andy was transferred to ICU, where he was intubated and placed on a ventilator. The symptoms advanced to paralysis of his entire body.

After a week or so, Andy was transferred back to the step-down unit, still on a ventilator, as he was unable to breath on his own.

Background:

Every morning, as the charge nurse on the step-down unit, I would make rounds with the residents and intensive care physician as well as the social worker, dietitian, physical therapist, and any other medical professionals involved with the patient's care. The primary nurse would also be present.

This day was a life-changing day for Andy--and for me.

All of the people involved in Andy's care were assembled in Andy's hospital room, including Andy's loving wife. The attending physician was not present. The resident led the group discussion.

This is close to how it went:

Fourth-Year Resident: "Hello. Mrs. Dufresne, you know that we have been unable to get your husband off of life support for many days. We don't think he will ever come off of the ventilator. Do you have any questions?"

Mrs. Dufresne: Audibly crying. I walked over to her, handed her Kleenex, and hugged her tightly.

Resident: After a few minutes: "Mrs. Dufresne, did you hear me? Do you understand what I just said?"

Mrs. Dufresne: Still sobbing. "Yes."

Resident: In front of Andy, who was awake on the ventilator: "Mrs. Dufresne, I recommend that you go ahead and make funeral arrangements."

Mrs. Dufresne: Sobbing louder.

Me: Staring at the resident angrily and holding up Mrs. Dufresne who felt like she was slipping down to the floor.

Andy: Tears flowing down his cheeks, looking horrified.

Me: Shaking in disgust: To the female resident doctor who I will rename Darth Vader: "Could you please step outside so that we can talk?"

I guided Mrs. Dufresne to a chair and told her and Andy that I would be back after speaking with the resident.

I left the room and guided Darth Vader to a private area so that we could talk.

Me: Yelling. "What the hell did you just do? I will tell you exactly what you just did. You walked into a patient's room and robbed the patient and his wife of hope. Hope is the most important thing that a patient has to hold onto. You are a resident who apparently thinks she is God. I am so angry at your arrogant behavior that I want to vomit. Now you go back to your attending physician and send him to me immediately before I blow a gasket!"

As a charge nurse, I usually did not have a patient assignment.

Nonetheless, I took the primary nurse aside and asked her if it was ok for me to be Andy's primary nurse from now on. She had no issue with my request. I immediately took over Andy's care.

I walked back into Andy's room and slammed the door shut. I took Mrs. Dufresne's hand and guided her over to her husband's bedside. The ventilator noise was in the background.

I wiped the tears from Andy's face. I tried to compose my thoughts as tears were racing down my face, as well.

Me: "Mr. and Mrs. Dufresne, I have taken over care of you, Andy. From now on, during the day shift, I will be your nurse until you walk out the front door of this hospital. Do you both understand me?"

Tears were flowing down Mrs. D. face.

Tears were flowing down Andys face.

Tears were flowing down my face.

Me: "Now then. I am going to get physical therapy, respiratory therapy, the primary doctor, and nutritional services together. We are going to formulate a plan of care for you today. We are officially starting your recovery this minute."

"You just need to do what we ask of you, Andy. I need you to participate in physical and occupational therapy. I need you to follow the dietitian's advice, once you are able to eat. I need you to take the medications that will be prescribed. Most importantly, Andy, I need you to wrap your brain around the fact that you are going to heal and walk out of here. This is the biggest war that you will ever fight in. You are not going to die. I am going to do everything I can to prevent that from happening. Do you understand?"

Andy blinked his eyes, as if to say yes, through all of his tears.

Me: "I need one promise from you, Andy. I need you to promise me that I will be present when you get out of this hospital. Is that clear? Even if I have to come over here on my day off, I want to witness this. Got it?"

Mrs. Dufresne hugged me and profusely thanked me.

We all cried louder, but this time with hope.

Andy came off of the ventilator within a few weeks. Within a month or two, he was able to walk with a walker. We would walk the halls together, even though he had been transferred to the med-surg unit once he came off of the ventilator.

I was present when he left the hospital and headed to a skilled nursing facility for more physical therapy and occupational therapy.

As God would have it, the skilled nursing facility was about a half a mile from my apartment building. My dog, Hershey, and I would take a walk and visit Andy, at least weekly. I would wheel Andy outside under a lovely tree. Hershey, my 20-pound mutt, would leap up onto Andy's lap, as if knowing Andy needed some lovin'. Andy loved Hershey and looked forward to his visits.

During that period of time, Andy informed me, over and over again, that he knew I was his guardian angel. In fact, he insisted on calling me "his angel" from then on. (More tears).

The Dufresnes kept in touch with me for years. They moved to Montana with their daughter, and they would send me yearly Christmas cards.

Andy passed peacefully in his '80s. I am certain that he left this planet knowing that a nurse's steadfast conviction in doing what was right, had saved his life, as he'd shared this sentiment with me for decades.

A nurse had changed the outcome of Andy's life. A nurse had been his advocate. A nurse had treated this stranger with compassion, as if he were a family member. A nurse had given Andy and his wife hope for the future.

I am a nurse.

Acknowledgements

First and foremost, I would like to acknowledge my sister and brother-in-law, Debbie Lichtman and Steve Ladd, for their tireless help with the editing of this book, for their suggestions with the artwork, and simply for their endless love.

I want to thank my parents, Esther and Gideon Lichtman, for instilling in me the love of reading.

I also appreciate four dear nurse friends who listened and encouraged me to accomplish my lifelong goal of telling my story. Much love to these members of the Fab Five: Julie Gustafson, Fizzy Lange, Michelle Sanders, and Diane Zieour. (I am number five.)

A special thanks to Rich Percy, my "computer guy." He is the reason this manuscript exists on my laptop and was able to jet back and forth to my publisher so efficiently. Otherwise, I would have had to count on our U.S. Postal Service and you know that this would have stalled production until the year 2050.

Amazon Publishing guided me through every step of the final process. A special thanks to the Sr. Project Manager Liz Pearsons, the Sr. Editor and Formatter Marrian Robin, and the amazing and talented Sr. Illustrator and Designer Edna Rebecca.

Finally, I wish to acknowledge all of the humans who unknowingly or knowingly contributed to my life and to this composition. Without all of you, this book would not have become a reality.